"COVID" COMPENSATION

RECLAIM WEALTH & HEALTH

LOST TO LOCKDOWNS & "VACCINES"

A GLOBAL MEDICAL & LAW SELF-HELP GUIDE

"COVID19"
HISTORY'S BIGGEST CONFIDENCE TRICK
WORLD'S FINEST SCIENTISTS & LAWYERS
REPORT SHOCKING TRUTH

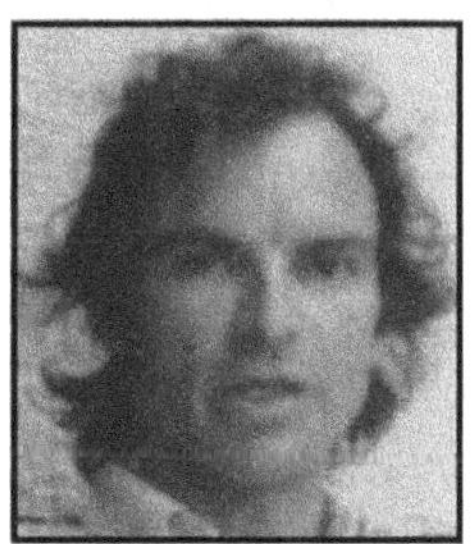

Lawrence Wolfe-Xavier

Editor for

CORONA ACCOUNTABILITY (Covid19) 2022

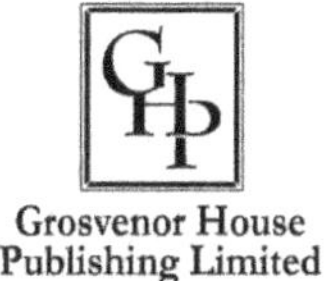

Grosvenor House
Publishing Limited

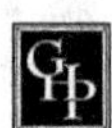

This book is published by
Grosvenor House Publishing Ltd
Link House
140 The Broadway, Tolworth, Surrey, KT6 7HT.
www.grosvenorhousepublishing.co.uk

A CIP record for this book
is available from the British Library

ISBN 978-1-80381-400-1
eBook ISBN 978-1-80381-401-8

CONTENTS

IMPORTANT NOTICE: WHY THIS BOOK WAS WRITTEN

This book was written primarily for the following reasons:

1. The Editor discovered during his research, that from March 2019 onwards, the Greatest Evil perpetrated against Humankind - nearly 8Bn people all over the world, by very few people say little more than 300, that Evil being "Covid19" and its machinations, was coming into play.
2. The Editor considers such Evil to be wrong and a violation of Natural Law.
3. It was further considered that these 8Bn people had a right to know of this Evil, particularly when Globalist Powers harnessed all the might of global mainstream media to prevent them from learning of it.
4. Furthermore, the people in control of the implementation of this Evil should be brought to account and to be brought to justice for their Evil.
5. The people on knowing the full Truth of this matter, would have in their hands a Global "COVID" Medical & Law Self-Help Guide, that would inform them of procedures and processes by which they may seek full medical, emotional and financial compensation.
6. The book would also inform the readers of medical solutions that would, at least in part using the best practices available, resolve their problems with "Covid19" and the "vaccines".

If you are any doubt as to the **extreme evil** under the cloak of "healthcare" that "Covid19" "vaccination" has been perpetrated by powerful, wealthy, and influential people against ordinary working people of whom the editor is one, please be informed that three litigation cases have commenced against **Bill Gates** of 'Bill and Melinda Gates Foundation' for **mass murder**. "Vaccines" will be part of the indictments.

Ref: Dr Reiner Fuellmich International Anti-Corporate Corruption Trial Lawyer (Germany/ USA) Cofounder 'Corona Investigative Committee' and Founder 'International Crime Investigative Committee' 'ICIC'- 5th October 2022

Ref: https://tntradiolive.podbean.com/e/reiner-fuellmich-on-the-shannon-joy-show-05-october-2022/

If any reader in the world thinks that he/she can rebut and/or refute the assertions of some of the finest independent minds in the world in virology, infectious diseases, pulmonary critical care, immunology, epidemiology, microbiology, medicine, law etc including two Nobel Prize winners and one Nobel prize nominee whose work is reported in this book, then

please do so via the website contact email address. Please ensure that you present your work with fully authenticated data driven actualities, not silly 'conspiracy theories' i.e. The CIA at their very best.
Website: https://covid19compensation2022.com/
Email: corona-accountability-covid19-2022@protonmail.com

A proportion of the royalties from the sales of this book will be used to help those less fortunate than others.

Lawrence Wolfe-Xavier Editor Corona Accountability (Covid19) 2022 Nov. 2022

HOW TO USE THIS SELF-HELP GUIDE, LEGAL NOTICES AND THE 'GREAT RESET'/'NEW WORLD ORDER' DANGERS THE MORAL ENIGMA OF THE 300 EVIL SLAVES

Note: Scientific Papers in this book refer to over 500 Global Citations

THE 'GREAT RESET'/'NEW WORLD ORDER' DANGERS

'***2030: You'll own nothing. And you will be happy. Whatever you want you'll rent***'

Quoted:

Klaus Schwab, Executive Chairman, World Economic Forum WEF

Ref: https://www.facebook.com/watch/?v=10153920524981479

THIS MEANS NO MORE PRIVATE OWNERSHIP FOR THE MANY!
YET EVEN MORE PRIVATE OWNERSHIP FOR THE "ELITE" FEW!
The many will rent from the "Elite" few and make them Even Richer,
Whilst they become Even Poorer! A Post-Industrial Feudalism.

The People of the world will NOT OWN: their own home, their garage, their own furniture, their garden, their curtains, their cars, their second home (if they have one), their electronic home entertainment equipment i.e., television, radio, record player; their mobile phones, laptops, tablets, their garden furniture, their DIY tools and equipment, their reading desk and lamp, their watch, jewellery, diary, pens and paper and toilet rolls!

'World's Richest 1 Percent Own Twice as Much as Bottom 90 Percent'

Quote

'Philanthropy News Digest'

Ref: https://philanthropynewsdigest.org/news/world-s-richest-1-percent-own-twice-as-much-as-bottom-90-percent

According to Klaus Schwab WEF's 'Great Reset' it is going to get a lot worse

THE 'GREAT RESET' DANGER
<u>'GREAT RESET' ACTIVITY TIMELINE</u>

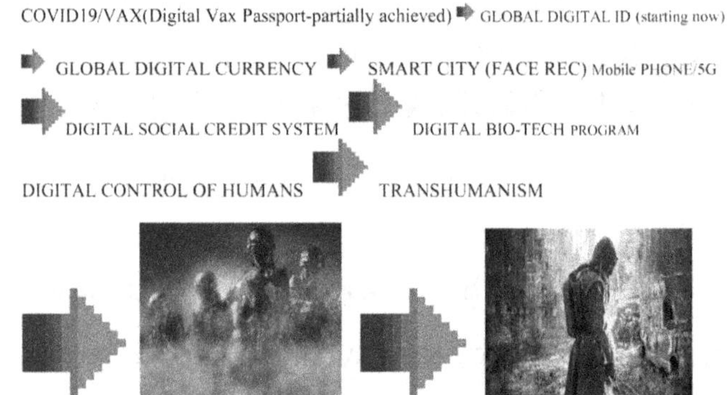

THE GLOBAL HUMANOID-ROBOT TOTALITARIAN DYSTOPIA

<u>Dr. Yuval Harari</u> advisor to Klaus Schwab WEF has endorsed this <u>insanity</u> on numerous occasions – see below:

Yuval Harari advisor to Klaus Schwab WEF World Economic Forum quote:

<u>'Governments and Corporations can hack Human Beings…you can manipulate them in ways that were previously impossible…. Soul, Spirit, Free Will - in humans, that's over!!!'</u>

Ref: **https://www.youtube.com/watch?v=NV0CtZga7qM**

Dr Reiner Fuellmich of the newly formed International Crimes Investigative Committee 'ICIC' (formerly Cofounder of the Corona Investigative Committee) describes the evil of 'The Great Reset' of the World Economic Forum WEF with quotes from the two leading persons, again: Klaus Schwab and Dr Yuval Harari:

https://www.onenewspage.com/video/20220917/14927553/Dr-Reiner-Fuellmich-Explains-The-Great-Reset-New.htm

The World Economic Forum WEF, under the Chairmanship of Klaus Schwab, who I would not employ even to run a whelk stall in Hartlepool, has under its "genius" a Young Global Leader Programme!! What does Harari and his side-kick Schwab know about running the world – they have never even run an ironmonger's shop! "Young" "Global" "Leaders" who have been "trained" by these WEF blockheads include Emmanuel Macron, Angela Merkel, Nicolas Sarkozy, Justin Trudeau (Trudy for short), and Tony Blair, Deontological Ethicists all! Apart from Blair who is a non-convicted war criminal, ref: Kofi Annan, Secretary General United Nations. None of them could run a whelk stall in Hartlepool either.

The 'Great Reset' threats to ordinary, hard-working people throughout the world needs no further explanation! This must be stopped.

The first explanation as to why these two blockheads, Schwab and Harari think that they believe in this nonsense is very, very simple indeed. It is very simple because these are two very simple "men". They are nothing more than 'materialists', they know nothing of life beyond the material because they never speak of it - even with their vast "erudition". They know nothing about Natural Law, Ontology, Metaphysics, Epistemology, Logic or most importantly Ethics; as stated, they are simple minded materialists.

The second reason relates to their states of "Mind". Dr Reiner Fuellmich since mid-2020, when this "Covid" cretinism and fracas started to move into full swing, has been researching this bizarre phenomenon with a global team of hundreds of lawyers and thousands of scientists – some of the finest independent minds in the world in their field. He has stated that on good authority, from the psychologists and psychiatrists whom he has been working with, that these two, who in the catalogue go as "men", are considered to be PSYCHOPATHS, MEGALOMANIACS AND SOCIOPATHS.

'Ay, in the catalogue ye go for men;
As hounds, and greyhounds, mongrels, spaniels, curs,
Shoughs, water-rugs, and demi-wolves, are 'clept
All by the name of dogs:..'

William Shakespeare 'Macbeth'

1. A psychopath is characterized by persistent antisocial behaviour, impaired empathy and remorse, and bold, disinhibited, and egotistical traits.
2. A megalomaniac is someone who has an unnaturally strong wish for power and control, or thinks that they are much more important and powerful than they really are.
3. A Sociopath refers to a pattern of antisocial behaviours and attitudes, including manipulation, deceit, aggression, and a lack of empathy for others.

In consideration that Harari has clearly, on numerous occasions, stated publicly:

'Governments and Corporations can hack Human Beings...you can manipulate them in ways that were previously impossible.... Soul, Spirit, Free Will - in humans, that's over!!!'

as shown above. Then the terms used above are particularly apt to describe Harari. They are also most fitting to describe Schwab, who comes across as a very cheap Bond film Mr Bad-Guy!

Under Natural Law these two "men" above show, based on statistical probability theory, to be examples of Natural Law anomalies. Natural Law is not perfect because it exists in Space and in particular, Time. Nothing that exists in space-time can be perfect because it is under the obligations of exterior, uncontrollable causality. Natural Law is hence not perfect but exists in *'An Imperfect Balance of Harmony of Being'*. © 2022 Lawrence Wolfe-Xavier

We now move onto statistics and probability. There is the natural phenomenon of Standard Deviation whereby any statistical data set will follow the diagram below. Where the vertical axis (y axis) is the specific value of an item in the data set and the horizontal axis (x axis) is the number of the particular item occurring. It does not matter what the data set is, it might be: degree grades in a class of students, height of oak trees of certain age, speed that a fast bowler in cricket can bowl a ball, the loudness of a species of domestic dog bark etc etc.

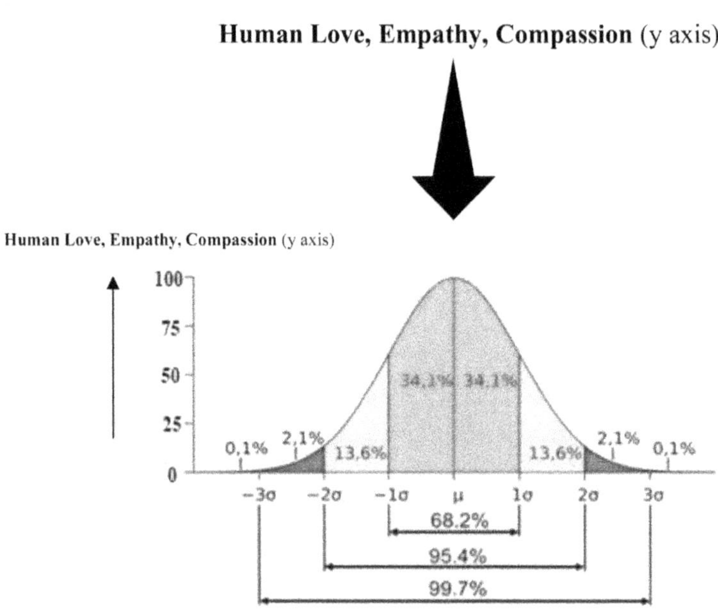

Human Population Percentage (x axis)

The diagram above is an indicative, generic one and the numerical scale on the y axis is not relevant to our discussion. What is relevant is the numerical distribution about the average. Whatever the y axis might be, the percentage of the number of the items in the x axis will be 68.2% within +1 and -1 standard deviation, 95.4% within -2 and +2 standard deviations, and almost 100% i.e., 99.7% within -3 and +3 standard deviations. In our example above we can observe the numerical distribution of those of us with Human Love, Empathy, Compassion about the average value.

At the extremes of minus and positive there are c. 0.1% in both cases. In terms of Human Love, Empathy, Compassion then those on the left i.e. – (minus) 0.1% might be considered to be those persons who are sadly very, very unwell, they perhaps even do not have any Human Love, Empathy, Compassion for themselves, let alone their fellow Humankind! These people are typically confined to institutions that try to help them as best they can.

At the + (positive) end of 0.1% these persons one might say, are perfectly conscious and perfectly conscious of their consciousness. However, their Human Love, Empathy, Compassion is as low as those confined to institutions. This is why they can "operate" on this mass murder programme level with little or no remorse. Such a concept as remorse is not within them, similarly neither is Human Love, Empathy, Compassion.

This is why they have no compunction regarding Evil, they have no concept of Evil. That is their problem. For the most part, certainly these idiots do, we have to live in society (despite what Margaret Thatcher may have thought that she believed) and this society, as are others such as Papua New Guinea tribesman, African Pygmies of The Congo etc., is bound by Moral and Legal Laws in order for it to function in any form of coherence, efficiency and efficacy.

These persons are obviating the Moral and Legal Laws by which they are supposed to operate. They are c. 300 persons or perhaps more, the remainder are 6Bn – I exclude China – those poor people live in the Mind of One Man! Heaven forbids! Or perhaps it doesn't!

The Moral Enigma of The 300 Evil Slaves

© 2022 Lawrence Wolfe-Xavier

It has been written, that since the beginning of Feudalism in 11th Century Europe, Europe and by default the rest of the world, has been essentially, completely ruled over by approximately thirteen blood line families. These families have a second tier of evil that supports them, shall we say there is a total of circa. 300 such evil people. It is the 300 Evil Slaves who are of interest to us. These people, as explained above, have no Human Love, Empathy, Compassion, these faculties are as low as those poor, unfortunate persons who are confined to 'learning difficulty' and other such institutions. This is why the Evil 300 slaves can "operate" on this mass murder programme level with little or no remorse. Such a concept as remorse is not within them, similarly neither is Human Love, Empathy, Compassion. This is their **Great Regret**! They are slaves to it – they are self-inflicted slaves to their own Evil. They live in a perverse reality where, what the majority of human beings have: Human Love, Empathy, Compassion – the very, very, inherent core of what it is to be Human; THEY DO NOT HAVE and they know it and they further know that THEY WILL NEVER HAVE IT! It is out of this profound recognition and deep regret that the Evil 300 do what they do. What they know they can NEVER HAVE, they seek to destroy. This is typical of such weaklings. They are psychopathically JEALOUS OF YOU, the Human All Too Human! Human all too Human is what you are and must strive to become better than what you are. The Imperfect Harmony of The Universe(s) will have its way with Evil 300 slaves. Why? Because they are violating what they have absolutely no knowledge of, The Imperfect Harmony of The Universe(s). Every single human being, mammal, creature, fish, invertebrate, tree, plant, flower and any and all other forms of life that becomes upon and within LIFE, by its creation through, and of, The Imperfect Harmony of The Universe(s) has a right to that LIFE. Indeed, its is its duty to fulfil that life for which it, and the Universe(s) are its purpose. [This concept will be expanded upon in subsequent writings.]

However, we the people, have the right to forbid these Evil people their Evil Intent and forbid them we must!

Ref: Alex Thomson - Expert Witness, [Corona Investigative Committee see Appendix I p44 – PDF Download File] former Officer of Britain's Signal Intelligence Agency: *'Yes. I have never found better material than that of a writing duo which is Dutch/German American. The Dutchman is Robin de Ruiter. His American German co-author is Fritz Springmeier from South Carolina. They have the rather shocking book titled* ***'Bloodlines of the Illuminati'****. But their work is solid.'*

[Please note that some passages in the book are repeated in differing chapters. This is because these passages are applicable to more than one chapter.]

Legal Notice A
LEGAL NOTICE

The contents of this book and its associated website contains material that **may be used in forthcoming criminal prosecutions worldwide**. Any persons or organisations tampering with this book or the website, the website content or its third-party URL links and their content may be liable to prosecution for **interfering with criminal case evidence**. This Notice is addressed to all persons including Big Tech Companies such as Google, Facebook, Twitter et al.

Legal Notice B
References in later Chapters

Dr Reiner Fuellmich – International Anti-Corporate Corruption Trial Lawyer – **Chairman Corona Investigative Committee** (Germany/World-Wide) Founder 'International Crime Investigative Committee' 'ICIC' and a world-renowned trial lawyer with almost three decades of experience in suing large fraudulent corporations, such as Deutsche Bank, Volkswagen, etc. **stated these "Covid19" "Vaccines" have been proven to be neither effective nor safe, but extremely dangerous and even lethal.**

His investigation serves as a model proceeding to secure indictments against some of the **criminally and civilly responsible figureheads of these "vaccine" "pandemic" crimes against humanity**, as listed below (Dr Fuellmich has named these listed below):

1. **Bill Gates Bill and Melinda Gates Foundation**
2. **Dr Fauci Chief Medical Advisor to President USA, Director of NIAID**
3. **Tedros Adhanom Ghebreyesus Director-General of the World Health Organization WHO**
4. **Dr Drosten Researcher/Designer of [worthless] PCR Tests** – Chapter 8
5. **Pfizer Pharmaceutical Corporation USA**
6. **Blackrock Investment Management Company USA**

Legal Notice C

A copy of this book including the Report (see Appendix I) will be sent to Baroness Hallett, the Chair of the UK Covid-19 Public Inquiry (June) 2022- so that she and her legal team may use its contents when undergoing the UK Covid-19 Public Inquiry. Three copies of the Report, continually being enlarged, were sent on 18th June 2022, 2nd August 2022 and 12th October 2022. Baroness Hallett's office responded confirming that the correspondence was on record at their office. See Appendix IV for the letter to Baroness Hallett that accompanied the copy of this book.

The replying Officer regarding the three copies of The Report was:

Abigail
Correspondence Team
UK Covid-19 Public Inquiry

Website: https://covid19.public-inquiry.uk/

Email: contact@covid19.public-inquiry.uk

Legal Notice D
References in later Chapters

In Australia, (suffered very severe lockdowns) good people are exposing this ruthless oppression.

Covid Inquiry 2.0 by Senator Malcolm Roberts, Australia - 16th August 2022

Referring to those responsible for the "SarCov2" "Covid19" "pandemic" lies:

Quotes:

'We will hound you down!'

'It has become clear, the people of this country* [Australia] *and globally have been steamrollered. It is also clear that it has been coordinated globally. It is also clear that it has been integrated not just over 6 months, not just over 2 ½ years, but it has been planned over decades. The changes to legislation in this country were done so that they could control doctors and the people.

***People are awakening and its thanks to Dr Altman and all the presenters here today. We know that this* ["SarCov2" "Covid19" "pandemic"] IS ALL BULLSHIT and we've been HAD.**

But we are going to hound you down. – you people who are guilty.

We will hound you down and hold you accountable and we will expose you globally, so that the people of Australia look forward to the future, because I love my kids and I'm looking forward to my grandkids.

We are going to save this country. Thank you.'

Senator Malcolm Roberts, Australia

Legal Notice E
References in later Chapters

No Government may Indemnify Breaches of Common, Civil or Criminal Law

No Government has the legal authority to indemnify Big Pharma and/or other distribution/implementation agents from effects of the "Covid19" "vaccines" for breaches of common, civil, or criminal law in the country providing the indemnity.

Please note below the civil and criminal prosecutions of some of Big Pharma.

Year	Company	Settlement	USA Laws violated
2012	GlaxoSmithKline	$3 billion ($1B criminal, $2B civil)	False Claims Act, FDCA
2009	Pfizer	$2.3 billion ($1.189B criminal)	False Claims Act, FDCA
2013	Johnson & Johnson	$2.2 billion	False Claims Act, FDCA

The Pfizer fine of $2.3 billion ($1.189B criminal) was the largest criminal fine in USA History for any offence! Would YOU indemnify a criminal company?

Ref: https://en.wikipedia.org/wiki/List_of_largest_pharmaceutical_settlements

Many leading scientific, medical, and legal world experts claim that there are many opportunities for the general public for: compensation, civil lawsuits, criminal lawsuits, foreseen complications and that the "vaccines" are really Bioweapons/Chemical Weapons and not true vaccines at all. A number of researchers have alluded to the "vaccines" being, in reality, "Bioweapons". This may be taken as a generic term for Bio/Chemical Weapons. However, Dr Wagh is emphatic when she describes them as Chemical Weapons as per her research studies into the "vaccines", see page 42, Appendix I p76 – PDF Download File.

Prof. Michel Chussodovsky - Professor of Economics

Quote:

'Covid19 'pandemic' [is the] *most serious social-economic crisis in History…'*
'Based on false statistics, 193 countries ordered to close down their economies...'
'the [Covid19] *'pandemic' is economic warfare…'* '[Pfizer] *"vaccines" programmes were homicide up to 28*th *February 2022, after that date,* [Pfizer] *had their data and therefore their "vaccines" programmes became murder…'*

Luc Montagnier, Nobel laureate in medicine for discovering HIV

Quote:

'These "vaccines" are poisons. They are not real vaccines. The mRNA [messenger RNA] *allows its message to be transcribed throughout the body, uncontrollably. No one can say for each of us where these messages will go. This is therefore a terrible unknown.'*

'The 3 vaccines Pfizer, AstraZeneca, Moderna contain a sequence identified by Information Technology as transformation into a prion. There is therefore a known risk to human health.'

Ref: **Luc Montagnier** was invited to the Luxembourg Parliament to accompany petitioners speaking out against compulsory "vaccination" on Wednesday 12th of January 2022. He spoke on the Covid "vaccines" and Geneticist Alexandra Henrion Caude was also there.

Ref: https://www.soulask.com/luc-montagnier-they-are-not-vaccines-they-are-poisons-speech-to-the-luxembourg-parliament/

Dr Michael McDowell

Quote:

'These* [Covid19] *vaccines have never been used on the human population before. They are tools of "Frankenstein Technology" a "mystery" concoction – a Bio-Weapon – the spike protein* [they contain] *is a pathogen and it will damage you.'

Ref: https://rumble.com/embed/vonrmq/

The UK government announced that it had granted Pfizer legal indemnity protecting the American pharmaceutical company from civil lawsuits due to any **unforeseen complications** arising from problems with its **"COVID-19 vaccine"**. The special legal indemnity was the result of an emergency government **consultation** in September 2020, when the UK Department of Health & Social Care determined that changes to civil liability were necessary to better facilitate the widespread use of a "COVID-19" "vaccine" in Britain.

Ref: https://www.jurist.org/news/2020/12/uk-government-grants-pfizer-civil-legal-indemnity-for-covid-19-vaccine/

Quote: ***'granted Pfizer legal indemnity protecting the American pharmaceutical company from civil lawsuits due to any unforeseen complications arising from problems with its COVID-19 vaccine'***

The key words here are: ***'civil lawsuits', 'unforeseen complications' and 'Covid-19 "vaccine"'.***

Legally, the word "vaccine" is very important, because the finest independent scientific minds in the world state that these products are not true vaccines. See Luc Montagnier and Dr Michael McDowell above. For full details see Chapters 6 and 7.

There is NO protection for: criminal lawsuits, foreseen complications nor "vaccines" that are Bioweapons/Chemical Weapons and not true vaccines at all. There is also no indemnity protection for breaking common or civil laws.

This Global "Covid" Medical & Law Self-Help Guide presents:

The Shocking Truth Revealed
by
The Finest Independent Scientific and Legal Minds in the World

Two Nobel Prize Winners: Luc Montagnier, Kary Mullis
One Nobel Prize Nominee: Dr Zelenko
The Most Cited Specialist in the World: Professor John P A Ioannidis
Architect of mRNA Technologies: Dr Robert Malone USA
Dr Mike Yeadon Dr Wagh Dr Blaylock Dr Fleming Dr McCullough Prof Bhakdi
Robert F Kennedy Jr – ex-president John F Kennedy's nephew – 'Big Pharma' Trial Lawyer
Dr Reiner Fuellmich – International Anti-Corporate Corruption Trial Lawyer – Chairman Corona Investigative Committee (Germany/World-Wide) Founder 'International Crime Investigative Committee' 'ICIC' etc. etc.

These leading world experts claim that there are many opportunities for compensation: civil lawsuits, criminal lawsuits, there were foreseen complications and that the "vaccines" are really Bioweapons/Chemical Weapons and not true vaccines at all!!

Luc Montagnier, Nobel laureate in medicine for discovering HIV

Quote (as above):

'These "vaccines" are poisons. They are not real vaccines. *The mRNA allows its message to be transcribed throughout the body, uncontrollably. No one can say for each of us where these messages will go. This is therefore a terrible unknown.'*

'The 3 vaccines Pfizer, AstraZeneca, Moderna contain a sequence identified by Information Technology as transformation into a prion. There is therefore a known risk to human health.'

The new regulation, Regulation 345 of the **Human Medicines Regulations of 2012**, prohibits civil liability against Pfizer or healthcare professionals distributing the vaccine for any damage that arises through use of the vaccine "in accordance" with its recommended use.

The Pfizer COVID-19 vaccine will, however, be scheduled alongside other vaccines subject to the **Vaccine Damage Payments Scheme**, which authorizes one-time payments of £120,000 for individuals who have been disabled in the rare case that a vaccine produces highly damaging side effects to patients. Such scheduling should allow claimants to still receive damages in the very unlikely event that they suffer serious side effects from the vaccine.

Legally, the word "vaccine" is very important, because the finest independent scientific minds in the world state that these products are not true vaccines. See Luc Montagnier and Dr Michael McDowell above. For full details see Chapters 6 and 7.

Ref: https://www.jurist.org/news/2020/12/uk-government-grants-pfizer-civil-legal-indemnity-for-covid-19-vaccine/

Please refer, in this Self-Help Guide to Chapters A, B and Chapters 1 to 14 and Chapter 18 for the thorough condemnation of what has taken place during this “Covid19” “pandemic”.

Legal Notice E

All of the evidence and advice provided in this book, including medical advice and legal advice is sourced verbatim from third parties of appropriate expertise and experience. It is provided in good faith for the education of the book’s readers so that the reader may make a better-informed judgment. If the reader is in any doubt, they should contact the source writer of the material directly. The sources are fully referenced throughout the book. The source writers are amongst the finest independent minds in the world in their field of expertise.

How to Use this Global “Covid” Medical & Law Self-Help Guide

If during the “Covid19” “pandemic” 2019-2022 onwards you have lost a loved one, lost income, lost your job, lost your business, had adverse “vaccine” side-effects, had adverse side-effects from masks, lockdowns and any other “covid19” mandated restrictions, then you may claim compensation.

This Self-Help Guide provides all of the relevant background information on “Sars-Cov2” and “Covid19” and the contact details of organisations that should be able to help you. Provide the organisations that you seek help from, with a copy of this book and explain to them your personal story. They will know the best approach for your personal circumstances.

Although this book was written from a UK perspective, the principles it covers are applicable to any country in the world subjected to “Sars-Cov2”/“Covid19” mandate restrictions. This Medical & Law Self-Help Guide may therefore be used by any person in any country affected by “Sars-Cov2”/“Covid19” Mandates – lockdowns, social distancing, masks etc.

Lawrence Wolfe-Xavier

CORONA ACCOUNTABILITY (Covid19) 2022 November 2022

ABOUT CORONA ACCOUNTABILITY (COVID19) 2022 ORGANISATION

A number of perceptive and aware individuals situated in various parts of the world, simultaneously perceived and understood, the significance of a number of huge incongruities in the "SarsCov2"/"Covid19" mainstream narrative. Communications between, and lengthy scientific studies commenced, among these persons.

Firstly, it was perceived in March 2020 that things did not 'add-up' regarding the news of "SarsCov2" and "Covid19". The "pandemic" emanated from a region of the world were democracy and truth are in no way obligatory. Indeed, the country has perhaps the worst record in the world regarding human rights violations. It has been known for some years that "viruses" do not hop from bats to humans. In a later chapter, Dr Richard Fleming states that in 2010 scientists in Wuhan, China KNEW that viruses in bats could NOT affect humans. Research proved this.

Secondly, yet the global blanket, in lockstep, propaganda narrative with not one single mainstream news outlet offering a scintilla of information that was in any microscopic way not finely tuned to the global one-dimensional false narrative pushed the view that the "Sars-Cov2" "virus" emanated from bats in a market in Wuhan, China.

All of the media, world-wide, reported exactly the same narrative as though they were ALL reading off the same script – which they were! This was very clear. Never before in history has the entire world media been in such homogenous uniformity on any particular singular issue. This global homogenous uniformity was particularly questionable in the light of this being a "novel" i.e., new "virus". Even supposedly independent, investigate journals, which have a reputation for truth and routing out corruption, followed the party line.

Thirdly, the "SarsCov2" "virus" had not been isolated prior to work commencing on so called "vaccines"! How is it possible to create a "vaccine" solution to a "virus" that has not been isolated and therefore the researchers have not a clue what the "virus" is constructed of and therefore cannot design a "vaccine" cure! "SarsCov2" even now almost 3 years after the outbreak in December 2019, has still not been isolated and it never will – see Chapters 1 and 2. Isolation is when there is no other matter within a specific sample other than the isolated virus itself. In this case, the correct term is in quotation marks, "virus" -, what has been called a "virus" is not a virus.

Fourthly, as in the third example above - the "SarsCov2" "virus" had not been isolated prior to work commencing on legislation such as UK Coronavirus Act 2020 and the implementation of so-called mandates – lockdowns, social distancing, masks etc. None of which had been properly scientifically investigated before their implementation. More importantly, how can it be lawful to create legislation in response to a "virus" when the "virus" has not been scientifically isolated, and its constituents identified? In reality it cannot. **The lawful validity of the UK Coronavirus Act 2020 is certainly open to challenge in a High Court.**

Fifthly, the companies creating the "vaccines" are hardly to be trusted. Big Pharma has been prosecuted practically continuously, for over a century of malpractice, for huge amounts of money! The Opioid Epidemic of 1911 onwards is just one example, with the Suffolk County v Purdue lawsuit in 2018. In 2007 Purdue Frederick Company Inc, an affiliate of Purdue Pharma, along with 3 company executives, pleaded guilty to criminal charges of misbranding.

Ref: https://en.wikipedia.org/wiki/Timeline_of_the_opioid_epidemic

Year	**Company**	**Settlement**	**USA Laws violated**
2012	GlaxoSmithKline	$3 billion ($1B criminal, $2B civil)	False Claims Act, FDCA
2009	Pfizer	$2.3 billion ($1.189B criminal)	False Claims Act, FDCA
2013	Johnson & Johnson	$2.2 billion	False Claims Act, FDCA

Ref: https://en.wikipedia.org/wiki/List_of_largest_pharmaceutical_settlements

Sixthly, many of the world's greatest minds in the subjects of virology, immunology, epidemiology, microbiology, medicine, law etc including two Nobel Prize winners made very serious allegations against world governments, Big Pharma, "Health" officials etc. using such terms as: **'mass murder', 'crimes against humanity', 'genocide'**. Words such as "mass murder, crimes against humanity, genocide" do not fall readily from such fine minds and serious intellects.

Ref: **Report** Grand Jury Appendix I p15 et al – PDF Download File, Dr Mike Yeadon Appendix I p14 et al – PDF Download File

Seventhly, eighthly, etc. etc. see book Chapters A, B, 1 to 14 and 18.

As consequence **CORONA ACCOUNTABILITY (Covid19) 2022 Organisation** was formed and this book was written.

ABOUT THE EDITOR

Lawrence Wolfe-Xavier

/Wit/Aphorist/Philosopher/Writer/Polemicist/Literary Historian/ /'Socratean' Dialectician/Photographer/Hunter/

Readers' quotes about the Author:

'Genius'

'An Exceptional Man.'

'A Warrior'

'High intellectual ability peppered with a profound spiritual intelligence is not a dish so common as one would hope. Lawrence Wolfe-Xavier has my respect.'

'I must say I admire the varieties of truth your courageous mind reveals...merci'

'Raw Intellect'

'Though this guy is on another level'

'Indeed, you remind me a lot of Oscar Wilde' [1854-1900]

'Very like Thomas Chatterton' [1752-1700]

He writes answers to questions on Intelligence, Genius, IQ, Philosophy, World Events, Literature, and other subjects on the Internet with more than 2M content views and with circa 40,000 readers per month. A 'most viewed' writer on many occasions.

Measured IQ 170/174 (SD 16) – Sigma Test, the most interesting and difficult un-timed, creative thinking, IQ Test in the world. Top 99.9996599% of global population.

ACKNOWLEDGEMENTS

Lawrence Wolfe-Xavier and CORONA ACCOUNTABILITY (Covid19) 2022 proffers their deepest thanks and gratitude to the following persons and organisations whose courageous, honest, and sublime work has made this book possible.

Vanessa, Lydia, Paul, Tom, Kevin – A Stand in The Park for all their hard work in helping with the Report in Appendix I.

Dr Reiner Fuellmich International Anti-Corporate Corruption Trial Lawyer (Germany/ USA) Cofounder 'Corona Investigative Committee' and Founder 'International Crime Investigative Committee' 'ICIC' https://icic.law/, 'Corona Investigative Committee' Grand Jury, Professor John P A Ioannidis, Kary Mullis, Dr Vladimir Zelenko, Dr Robert Malone USA, Dr Mike Yeadon, Dr Wagh, Dr Blaylock, Dr Fleming, Dr McCullough, Dr Michael McDowell, Dr. Pierre Kory, Prof Bhakdi, Dr Katrina Reiss, Dr. Simone Gold, Luc Montagnier, Nobel laureate in medicine for discovering HIV, Robert F Kennedy Jr – ex-president John F Kennedy's nephew – 'Big Pharma' Trial Lawyer, Dr Richard Fleming, Baruch Vainshelboim – Stanford Mask Study; Dr. Jay Bhattacharya, Dr. Sunetra Gupta and Dr. Martin Kulldorff – Great Barrington Declaration, The New England Journal of Medicine, Dr. Astrid Stuckelberger, N. Ana Garner, Prof. Michel Chussodovsky, Dr Francis Boyle, Torsten Engelbrecht, Konstantin Demeter, Dr Christian Anderson, Christine Massey, https:// www.ellaster.nl/ Ellaster.nl, Dr Elens, Doctor Joseph Mercola, Dr. John Coleman, Andreas Kalcker, Dr. Tom Cowan, Harry Vox, Dr Wuzunyou, Dr. Sona Pekova, Dr. Immanuel, Prof. Dr. Ulrike Kammerer, Professor Didier Raoult, Dr. Rob Elens, Dr Wuzunyou, Dr Richard Fleming, Dr. Carrie Madej, Thomas Renz, Dr David John Sorenson – stopworldcontrol. com, Dr Altman, Stew Peters, Anthony Patch, Matthew Skow, Project Veritas, https://www. icandecide.org/, Nicholas Stumphauzer, Brownstone Institute, Geert Vanden Bossche, Dr Vernon Coleman, John O'Looney, University of San Francisco, Salk Institute, Pieter Borger, Bobby Rajesh Malhotra, Clare Craig, Lazarus Report, Kevin McKernan, Klaus Steger, Paul McSheehy, Lidiya Angelova, Fabio Franchi, Thomas Binder, Henrik Ullrich, Makoto Ohashi, Stefano Scoglio, Marjolein Doesburg-van Kleffens, Dorothea Gilbert, Rainer Klement, Ruth Schruefer, Berber W. Pieksma, Jan Bonte, Bruno H. Dalle Carbonare, Kevin P. Corbett, Ulrike Kämmerer, Dr. Sona Pekova, Prof. Dr. Ulrike Kammerer, Dr. Heiko Schoening, Senator Malcolm Roberts – Australia, Brian Rose – London Real TV, Dr Dolores Cahill, Dr Rashid Buttar, Dr Judy Mikovits, David Icke, Tim Gielen, Dr. Denis G. Rancourt, Jane Doe, Paul Elias Alexander, Dr. Scott Atlas, Dr. Robert Young, The Informed Consent Action Network (ICAN), La Quinta Columna researchers, Eran Bendavid, Fritz Springmeier, Christopher Oh, Jay Bhattacharya, Simone Gold, M.D., J.D, America's

Frontline Doctors, EudraVigilance, Daryl Brown - The No Corruption Alliance, American Institute for Economic Research, Geza Tarjanyi, Dr. Jane Ruby, Vittorio Sgarbi, Dr. Elke de Klerk, Dr Sam White, Doctors for Information, Doctors for Truth, World Doctors Alliance, World Freedom Alliance, Alex Thomson, Dexter L-J. Ryneveldt, Jonathan Sumption - Justice of the Supreme Court UK, Patrick King (v The Crown, UK), Peter Wood, Carlo Maria Vigano, Zach Vorhies, Udo Ulfkotte, Dr. Brian Tyson, Dr. Stella Immanuel, Dr. David Brownstein, Dr. Joseph Mercola, Dr. Richard Bartlett, Prof. Dan Nicolau, Dr. Jeffrey Barke, Ricardo Delgado, La Quinta Colmuna, Josep Pàmies, Elizabeth Lee Vliet, MD, Robin de Ruiter, Dr. Francis Boyle, Mike Adams, The Hardwick Alliance for Real Ecology (HARE), Leslie Manookian, Michael O'Bernicia, Christina Figueres, Bjorn Pirrwitz, Dr. Naomi Wolf, Prof. Dr. Christian Kreiss, Dr Charles Hoff, Catherine Austin-Fitts, Professor Richard Werner, James Bush, Dipali Ojha, Dr. Shankara Chetty, Debbie Evans, Deana Pollard Sacks, Professor Robert West, Deanna McCleod, Dr Bryan Ardis, Dr Scott Youngblood, Dr Alexandra Henrion Caude, Dr. James Thorpe

https://www.bitchute.com https://londonreal.tv/

https://odysee.com/ https://awarriorcalls.com/

https://www.brighteon.com/ https://rumble.com/

https://www.thebernician.net/ www.delingpole.podbean.com

World Freedom Directory:

https://stopworldcontrol.com/map/?inf_contact_key=9f12092b3639c319a181287dcd1ea45309c74070ac2bf3cfa7869e3cfd4ff832

NOTE TO THE READER

You have been deliberately lied to, the world over, in the most evil of ways. The lies have been orchestrated at a high, trans-global level, beyond the powers of nation states and using control over governments, the media, the "scientists" and the people. **If you have been fooled, it is not your fault.** The propaganda was so vast and so intensive that most people, the world over, were fooled. Now, two and half years after the start of the "Covid pandemic" around December 2019, **the TRUTH is revealed**. Now your day has come. **Now your just compensation can be realised**.

Dr. Mike Yeadon, former Vice President, Head of Respiratory Health, Pfizer Pharmaceuticals (UK) quote: ***'we contend that all the main narrative points about the "coronavirus" named 'SARS-CoV-2' are lies. Furthermore, all the 'measures' imposed on the population are also lies.'***

The CORONA ACCOUNTABILITY (Covid19) 2022 organisation can barely believe that it has been obliged to write this book; but it has!

On publication, copies of this book will be sent to some of the UK Authorities and individuals listed below requesting them, under The Freedom of Information Act 2000, to **provide copies of documentation that refute and rebut the very serious allegations of Mass Murder, Crimes against Humanity, Genocide contained in this book.** Very serious allegations made by from the world's finest independent minds in virology, immunology, epidemiology, microbiology, medicine, law etc including two scientific Nobel Prize winners and one scientific Nobel prize nominee:

Recipient	**Office** (at the time – 2019/2020 onwards)
Boris Johnson	**Prime Minister**
Matt Hancock	**Health & Social Care**
Nadhim Zahawi	**"Covid" "Vaccine" Deployment**
Michael Gove	**Cabinet Office**
Sajid Javid	**Health & Social Care**
Suella Braverman	**Attorney General**
Priti Patel	**Home Office**
Baroness Hallett	**Chair Covid Inquiry 2021-**
Christopher Whitty	**Chief Medical Officer/Chief Medical Advisor**
Patrick Vallance	**Chief Scientific Advisor**

June Munro Raine	**CEO MHRA** - Medicines and Healthcare Products Regulatory Agency
Charlie Massey	**CEO GMC** – General Medical Council
Amanda Pritchard	**CEO NHS** – National Health Service
Neil Ferguson	**Researcher** - Imperial College, London

All of the information provided by these persons and authorities under The Freedom of Information Act 2000 as requested will be published on the website: https://covid19 compensation2022.com/ within 48 hours of it being received.

No matter where you reside: USA, Canada, Germany, Italy, Spain, Australia or wherever in the world; you may send a copy of this book to your equivalent representatives to the list above, and ask for their refutations and rebuttals to the allegations made by the world's finest independent minds in virology, immunology, epidemiology, microbiology, medicine, law etc including two Nobel Prize winners that are littered all over this book. If you have in your country, a Freedom of Information Act or similar, you may request the recipients for their refutations and rebuttals to the allegations from the documents available under your 'Freedom of Information ACT'.

Please inform, via email, the CORONA ACCOUNTABILITY (Covid19) 2022 organisation of any successes that you may have achieved in reclaiming your Health and Wealth and they will be documented on the website to help others to do the same.

Email: corona-accountability-covid19-2022@protonmail.com

Website: https://covid19compensation2022.com/

Contemporary History, from December 2019 to present (2022), must not be ignored.

The global suffering from "Sars-Cov2/Covid19" that has been unnecessarily inflicted on the world's population, by an elusive, ostensibly inhumane "elite", is so deplorable there are no words to describe it. It must be recorded for History, so that History may be their Judge. It must be without question, the greatest Human-to-Human unnecessarily, inflicted suffering and folly in the entire History of homo sapiens. Those who have suffered so unnecessarily and pointlessly must have their just compensation.

The global population has lost loved ones, lost businesses, lost income, suffered severe illnesses – both mental and physical, lost schooling, incurred massive inflation and most probably a prolonged recession to come. The global population has been subjected to the most horrible deprivation of natural human rights that men and women have lost their lives in achieving and protecting over centuries and centuries. All of this to no avail. It was all so unnecessary!

The global population should not blame themselves. They have been subjected to a most sophisticated, intense, rigourous and total black-out propaganda of a false narrative. No critical analysis has been permitted. All alternative narratives have been labelled "conspiracy theories" and relegated to suppressed non-mainstream social media outlets and have been dismissed by very dubious and false "fact checkers".

Only now, after years of intensive analysis, this book will reveal the TRUTH about "Sars-Cov2/Covid19" with testimonies from the world's finest independent minds.

Testimonies are presented verbatim by two Nobel Prize winners – one the inventor of the PCR Test in 1987/1988, the other the discoverer of HIV, a Nobel prize nominee – the inventor of a working remedy for "Covid19" using a combination of hydroxychloroquine, azithromycin, and zinc which was banned by the governments, medical authorities and the mass media, the architect of mRNA methodologies now personally banned from 'Twitter', Robert F Kennedy – ex-president John F Kennedy's nephew - a 'Big Pharma' trial lawyer, Prof. John Ioannidis, Professor of Medicine (Stanford Prevention Research), of Epidemiology and Population Health, Stanford University USA – the most widely cited expert person in the world in this field. Corona Accountability (Covid19) 2022 has no Nobel prize winners or other such specialist experts on its staff to check the data validity of every single research paper referenced, nor does any professional journal such as 'The Lancet'; therefore the data-driven views of these leading world experts are presented verbatim and in good faith for educational purposes and Corona Accountability (Covid19) 2022 has no reason to doubt the veracity of the data and conclusions provided, thus carries no liability. If the reader requires further information, it may be wise to approach each associated expert directly.

All of the above and thousands of other technical experts worldwide and hundreds of lawyers worldwide rigourously refute the main narrative of the "Sars-Cov2/Covid19" "pandemic" and rebut the validity of all of its major consequences.

This book is their story. This book is your story.

November 2022

p.s.
If there is any person or organisation in the world who/that can legitimately refute any of the allegations by these world leading experts, then please do so by writing to:

corona-accountability-covid19-2022@protonmail.com

Your Genius will respectfully be published world-wide, provided that the research data supplied, irrefutably backs up any claim made.

"For the Power of Truth is incredibly Great and of Unutterable Endurance."

Arthur Schopenhauer
'The World as Will and Representation'
'Second Book: The World as Will. First Aspect'

'If you have no Fear of Death, which you have no reason to; you have no Fear of Anything.'

'One Person alone, cannot change the World in its Entirety; but one Person's Idea can change the World Entirely.'

Lawrence Wolfe-Xavier

INTRODUCTION

Do not be concerned that you may have been fooled. <u>You are not alone</u>. Just over 75% of the UK population have been fooled by the biggest, most intensive, global propaganda campaign in the History of the World. The majority of people all over the world have been fooled – in excess of 60%! Do not be concerned that you may have been fooled. **<u>You will be able to claim your compensation</u>.**

Let's do a simple test:

Type into your browser (Google etc) on your mobile phone, tablet or laptop the following:

382200 export 2017

382200 is one of the global product codes for the PCR Medical Test Kits as defined by WITS (**World Bank**) World Integrated Trade Solution. The figures (November 2022) state that the top global 5 exporters in 2017 were:

USA exported 6.57US$Bn, EU exported 6.36US$Bn, Germany exported 4.25US$Bn Netherlands US$1.96Bn, UK 1.78US$BN – all in 2017!

Note the URL link:

Ref: https://wits.**worldbank.org**/trade/comtrade/en/country/ALL/year/2017/tradeflow/Exports/partner/WLD/nomen/h5/product/382200

The WITS database comes under the auspices of <u>THE WORLD BANK</u>!

Then type in:

382200 import 2017

Scroll down the tables displayed, for both '382200 export 2017' and '382200 import 2017' and you will observe that practically the entire world circa 195 countries were in the business of exporting and importing PCR Medical Test Kits in 2017!!

The first outbreak of "Covid19" was announced by the World Health Organisation 'WHO' on 31st December 2019. Assuming that to have this huge amount of PCR Test Kits available for export in 2017, they would have to be designed/defined in say 2015, then manufactured in 2016. **This would mean that PCR Test Kits were first being conceived in 2015 a full 5 years before the WHO announced the "virus"!! How does that make sense?!**

Here is an explanation:

Representatives from c. 195 countries – the entire world – did not convene in a football stadium or other building suitably sized to accommodate all of them, (all with little designatory country flags to distinguish one from another) and discuss the whys and wherefores of how to globally initiate, specify, design, approve, manufacture, and **cross export and import** to every country in the world, internationally recognised and approved PCR Medical Test Kits all commencing at exactly the same time in 2017!

Ref: https://wits.worldbank.org/trade/comtrade/en/country/ALL/year/2017/tradeflow/Exports/partner/WLD/nomen/h5/product/382200

The complexity of the logistics of this enormous global exercise is not to be underestimated. All of these exporters have to produce "Covid" PCR Test Kits that satisfy the local individual Health and Safety guidelines of all the individual countries they export to! For this to work and it obviously did, the only way would be that this was NOT organised at the sovereign state national level. This is simply not feasible or believable. This process must have been meticulously planned and organised at a pan-global level, at a level of authority that was above that of sovereign national state governments. The only organisations that have that global power and reach are (plus possibly a few others less well known):

United Nations 'UN'
World Bank
World Health Organisation 'WHO'
World Economic Forum 'WEF'

All controlled and coordinated by the Evil300 under whom the UN, World Bank, WHO,WEF etc are merely puppets.

As you are no doubt aware, businesses world-wide use sophisticated market intelligence metrics to ascertain the risk involved in developing and bringing to market a new product. They only bring to market products that pass their stringent risk assessments. How can it possibly be, that the entire world of business agreed, (individually or together) at the same time, that the PCR Medical Test Kits passed their stringent market risk assessment? **The short answer was that no risk assessment was required!** This is possibly the first time in History that such a complex, multifarious, country inter-dependent, global project has taken place without the requirement for any risk assessment whatsoever!

This baffling fact was discovered by someone on **September 5, 2020**, who posted it on social media. It went viral all over the world. The next day, on **September 6,** the WITS suddenly changed the original product label 'COVID-19' into the vague term 'Medical Test Kits'. But their cover-up came too late: this critical information was uncovered and is being revealed by millions worldwide. In this case the product code was not 382200 but 300215, there was more than one product code for very similar, almost identical, products.

See diagram table below:

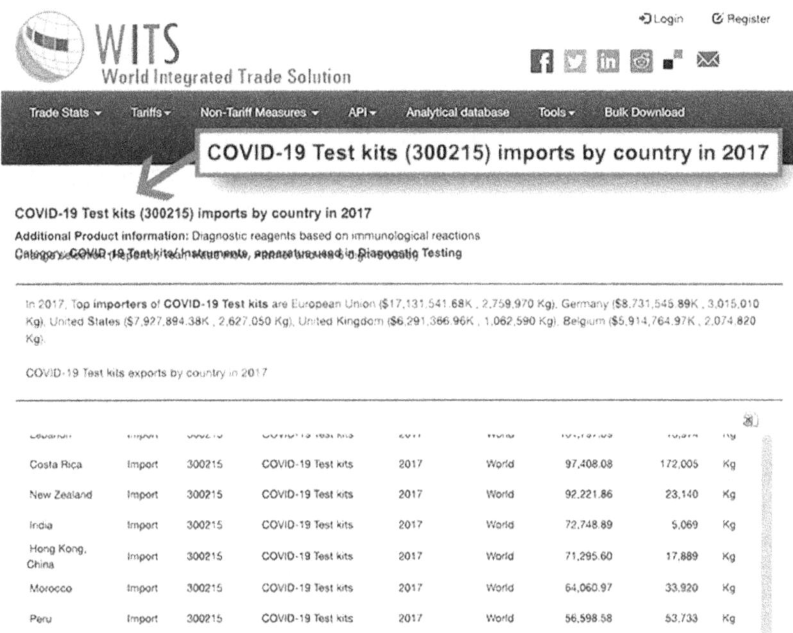

COVID-19 Test kits (300215) imports by country in 2017

Additional Product information: Diagnostic reagents based on immunological reactions

Category: COVID-19 Test kits/ Instruments, apparatus used in Diagnostic Testing

In 2017, Top **importers** of **COVID-19 Test kits** are European Union ($17,131,541.68K , 2,759,970 Kg), Germany ($8,731,545.89K , 3,015,010 Kg), United States ($7,927,894.38K , 2,627,050 Kg), United Kingdom ($6,291,366.96K , 1,062,590 Kg), Belgium ($5,914,764.97K , 2,074,820 Kg).

COVID-19 Test kits exports by country in 2017

Costa Rica	Import	300215	COVID-19 Test kits	2017	World	97,408.08	172,005	Kg
New Zealand	Import	300215	COVID-19 Test kits	2017	World	92,221.86	23,140	Kg
India	Import	300215	COVID-19 Test kits	2017	World	72,748.89	5,069	Kg
Hong Kong, China	Import	300215	COVID-19 Test kits	2017	World	71,295.60	17,889	Kg
Morocco	Import	300215	COVID-19 Test kits	2017	World	64,060.97	33,920	Kg
Peru	Import	300215	COVID-19 Test kits	2017	World	56,598.58	53,733	Kg

Ref: https://stopworldcontrol.com/2017-covid19-testkits.pdf

If you now google '300215 import 2017' you will see that the nomenclature COVID-19 TEST KITS has changed to 'MEDICAL TEST KITS' as we saw with product code 382200. Product codes 382200 and 300215 are presumably similar products although differing in some way. Fortunately for history, stopworldcontrol.com has saved and published this fact.

The detailed explanation for this very odd phenomenon will be explained in later chapters of this book.

The global power, control and falsely inflicted fear caused the majority of people in UK and the world to receive "vaccines" that had **not undergone full clinical trials** and that were **rushed to market in a matter of a year or so**. True vaccines typically take 7 to 10 years to bring to market using rigorous testing and full clinical placebo group trials. **The "Covid19" "vaccines" appeared on the market in a matter of 11 months.** The 'WHO' announced the "virus" to the public on 31st December 2019, the UK Government released "vaccines" to the public on 8th December 2020 a total of 11 months later. These "vaccines" have never undergone full clinical trials so the unsuspecting public allowed Pfizer – a proud Corporation, owner of the largest ever fine for criminal activities for anything in USA (see Ref below) - to inject into their bodies **experimental substances** that they knew nothing of, and therefore did not, and could not, provide **"informed consent"(a legal obligation)** and thereby became an unsuspecting new global 'breed' of 'human-guinea pigs' as part of a huge, global "vaccine" experiment. **The entire unsuspecting world population was unknowingly subjected to the largest human "vaccination" experiment in the History of the World.**

In 2009 Pfizer was the biggest criminal in the History of USA if you denote "biggest" by the size of the criminal and civil fines imposed upon the Company, being 2.3US$Bn for fraudulent marketing of which **1.189US$Bn was a criminal fine**; quote USA Justice Department ***'the largest criminal fine ever imposed in the United States for any matter.'***

Ref: https://www.justice.gov/opa/pr/justice-department-announces-largest-health-care-fraud-settlement-its-history

Furthermore, the global population was never in a position to provide informed consent for the "vaccinations" because the companies that produced them: Pfizer, Moderna, AstraZeneca, Johnson & Johnson etc. did not release the formulation of the "vaccines". It is only now after serious research by independent bodies that it can be revealed that the "vaccines" and the "Sars-Cov2" "virus" are both Bioweapons/Chemical Weapons produced in highest security Biosafety level 4 (BSL-4) bio-weapon labs. All of this meticulously planned global folly is fully explained in the subsequent chapters.

CHAPTER A

BRIEF HISTORY OF "SARS-COV2/COVID19"

'This is a <u>designed</u> human tragedy of Biblical proportions.'

Robert F Kennedy Jr Attorney at Law USA
Big Pharma Trial Attorney USA
Nephew of John F Kennedy - past President USA

The world was informed of the "Sars-Cov2/Covid19" outbreak with the first reported case in Wuhan, China. The first "Covid19" case was reported on December 8, 2019 (the first date of symptom onset based on the patients' recall during the investigation), in Wuhan City, the provincial capital of Hubei Province in Central China.

Consequently, in early 2020 and the following months there was a **world-wide 'nightmare'** that no one seemed to fully understand. This nightmare was known variously as "Coronavirus" "Sars-Cov2" and "Covid19". Coronaviruses are a group of viruses belonging to the family of Coronaviridae, which infect both animals and humans. Human coronaviruses can cause mild disease similar to a common cold, while others cause more severe disease. "Sars-Cov2" - Severe acute respiratory syndrome coronavirus 2 (SARS-CoV-2) was a "novel" (new) severe acute respiratory syndrome coronavirus. It was the name given to the particular "virus" found in Wuhan, China in 2019 and "Covid19" was the name of the illness that was supposedly caused by "Sars-Cov2".

Mass Induced Nightmare

The **nightmare** had only just begun and was to last almost two full years – 2020-2022. Horrible images appeared from China (not the most democratic country in the world) then from Italy and other countries until world-wide. Preposterous projections of not to happen global deaths based on very flawed computer models were bandied about like children's toffees to an unknowing mass of a very frightened and unfortunately deliberately ill-informed global population. Global mass media fanned the flames morning, day and night for many months on end. Inappropriate quarantine measures were globally, in lockstep, imposed that restricted human movement to an inhuman level that people were not permitted to see their loved ones when their loved ones were dying in hospitals and care homes! The world was a surreal, dystopian horror story – police vans patrolling the street, complete lockdown and no one allowed outside except for one hours walk, no gatherings greater than six, empty streets, closed and boarded shops, empty parks and empty beaches. Draconian civil rights restrictions were imposed. The severest on hard earned civil rights since World War II. The Global economic and social life the world over were about to fall into total collapse. On what data were these extreme measures taken? Was the world really under such a massive threat that we had to close down global capitalism for 2 years? The first time in World History that global feudalism, mercantilism or capitalism was closed for business. Had the benefits of these very severe measures been adequately assessed against the damage that they would also no doubt cause to the global economy and to individual person's lives throughout the world?

According to John P. A. Ioannidis – the most cited expert in the world in his field, it would appear not!

John P. A. Ioannidis - Physician Scientist Stanford University USA – most cited expert in the world in this field.

Quote:

'Acknowledging residual uncertainties, the available evidence suggests average global IFR* [Infection Fatality Ratio] *of~0.15%'

Ref: 2b page xx in The Report

The fatality rate of "Covd19" was c. 0.14% much the same as the common flu! Yet the world went mad! **Totally MAD!**

This restrictive madness was instigated in China, with Wuhan and five other cities completely isolated (locked down) from the rest of the world, these six cities were encircled by the army! China set the stage for how the world should respond to this "virus". The world dutifully and blindly followed. However, official China statistics reported, at the end of the "pandemic", that about 83,000 people were infected and fewer than 5,000 fatalities, a very, very small number in a country of 1.4Bn inhabitants.

Ref: 'Corona False Alarm? Facts and Figures' (publ. 2020) Dr Katrina Reiss Dr Sucharit Bhakdi pp 9,12

How dangerous was the "new killer virus"?

Gauging the true threat that the "virus" posed was initially impossible. Right from the beginning, the global media and politicians spread a distorted and misleading picture based on very fundamental flaws in data acquisition and especially on medically incorrect definitions laid down by the World Health Organisation (WHO), the Director-General is Dr. Tedros Adhanom Ghebreyesus.

Note: THE HAGUE, DEC. 1, 2020, 5 PM GMT+1 – A criminal complaint filed today with the International Criminal Court prosecutor charges the director-general of the World Health Organization, Dr. Tedros Adhanom Ghebreyesus, with responsibility for genocide and crimes against humanity as a top Ethiopian official before leading the WHO.

Ref: https://moneybloodandconscience.com/press-release/

Each positive laboratory test for the "virus" was to be reported as a "Covid19" case irrespective of clinical presentation. This definition represented an unforgivable breach of a first rule in infectiology; the necessity to differentiate between **"infection"** (invasion and multiplication of an agent in a host) and **"infectious disease"** (infection with ensuing disease). "Covid19" is the designation for severe illness that occurs only in about 10% of infected individuals, but because of incorrect designation, the number of "cases" surged and the "virus" vaulted to the top of the list of existential threats to the world. **Which it was not!**

Another serious mistake intended or otherwise, was that every deceased person (dead) who had tested positive for the "virus" entered the official records as a "coronavirus" victim.

This method of reporting violated ALL international medical guidelines!

The absurdity of giving "Covid19" as the cause of death in a patient who dies of cancer needs no comment. Nor does the greater absurdity of giving "Covid19" as the cause of death in patients who die of a road traffic accident with broken bones throughout their bodies, the remains of which were exotically tattooed by car tyre marks. [Ignore the facts when you need to bump up the "Covid19" fake numbers. This will be fully explained in later chapters.]

Correlation does not imply causation. Neither does utter stupidity, for that matter!

A False Catastrophe

This was a causal fallacy [deliberate?] that was destined to drive the world into a catastrophe. Truth surrounding the "virus" remained enshrouded in a tangle of rumours, myths and beliefs – deliberately ferociously driven by fear.

A French study, published on 19th March 2020 'Sars-Cov2 Fear versus Data', brought the first light into the darkness. Two cohorts of approximately 8,000 patients were grouped according to whether they were carrying everyday coronavirus or the "Sars-Cov2" "virus". Deaths in each group were registered over two months. However, the number of fatalities did not significantly differ in the two groups and the conclusion followed that the danger of "Covid19" was probably overestimated. [It most certainly was.]

In a subsequent study, the same team compared the mortality associated with respiratory viruses during the colder months of 2018-2019 and 2019-2020 (week 47-week 14) in south-eastern France. Overall, the proportion of respiratory virus-associated deaths among hospitalised patients was not significantly higher in 2019-2020 ("Covid19" first year) than the year before. Thus, the addition of "Sars-Cov2" to the spectrum of viral pathogens did not affect the mortality in patients with respiratory disease, i.e. "Sars-Cov2/Covid19" did not create a significant increase in mortality and all of the measures: Lockdowns, social distancing, masks etc were little more than a waste of time and resources, as fully explained in later chapters.

Ref: 'Corona False Alarm? Facts and Figures' (publ. 2020) Dr Katrina Reiss Dr Sucharit Bhakdi pp 15-16

Regrettably such voices of reason went unheard by our politicians. Neil Ferguson, Imperial College, London, made the headlines (but not much else?) when he stated that if nothing is done and the "virus" allowed to spread uncontrolled, more than 500,000 people will die in UK and 2 million in USA. Not only did this make the rounds, it struck fear into hearts and souls. [Was that the intention?]

Incidentally, Ferguson is the same authority who predicted 136,000 deaths due to mad cow disease (BSE), 200 million deaths due to avian flu and 65,000 deaths due to swine flu – in all cases they were ultimately a few hundred. In other words, he was wrong every time; very, very wrong! Do journalists actually have a conscience and, if so, why do they not check the facts before distributing their "news"? Naturally, here too it later became apparent that Ferguson's prediction was totally wrong. But this was never reported in the media.

Ref: 'Corona False Alarm? Facts and Figures' (publ. 2020) Dr Katrina Reiss Dr Sucharit Bhakdi

It is interesting to note here that Imperial College, London received donations for research from 'The Bill and Melinda Gates Foundation' of US$70M in c. 2020 and US$130M in the years leading up to 2020. Bill Gates pathological and dangerous obsession with vaccinating the entire world is well known, as is the vast amounts of money and power accrued from doing so. Gates is banned from India and Indian authorities are currently implementing his prosecution.

Because of this scientifically and medically dangerous erroneous situation a group of three concerned Doctors wrote the Great Barrington Declaration to bring the world's attention to the impending catastrophe.

Great Barrington Declaration

An approach we call Focused Protection.

Great Barrington Declaration

'As infectious disease epidemiologists and public health scientists we have grave concerns about the damaging physical and mental health impacts of the prevailing COVID-19 policies and recommend an approach we call Focused Protection.'

How did the Great Barrington declaration come about?

Why was the Declaration written?
The Declaration was written from a global public health and humanitarian perspective, with special concerns about how the current "COVID-19" strategies are forcing our children, the working class, and the poor to carry the heaviest burden. The response to the pandemic in many countries around the world, focused on lockdowns, contact tracing and isolation, imposes enormous unnecessary health costs on people. In the long run, it will lead to higher "COVID" and non- "COVID" mortality than the focused protection plan we call for in the Declaration.

Who is the intended audience?
This is an international declaration, written with concerns for the entire world. It was written for the public, fellow scientists, and government officials.

Who wrote the Declaration?
The Declaration was written by Dr. Jay Bhattacharya, Dr. Sunetra Gupta and Dr. Martin Kulldorff. A family member and a journalist helped with phrasing, grammar, and proof reading. Nobody else saw the declaration before it was completed in its final form.

When was the Declaration written, signed and released?
The Declaration was written from October 2 to October 4, 2020. It was signed on October 4, after which it was sent to scientific colleagues. It was released to the public on October 5, 2020.

Who initiated the Declaration?
Dr Kulldorff invited Dr Bhattacharya and Dr Gupta to Massachusetts to record a video outlining an alternative to the current "COVID-19" strategy. While meeting, the three spontaneously decided to also write a short Declaration to summarize the thinking.

Why was the Declaration signed in Great Barrington?
The Declaration was written and signed at the American Institute for Economic Research, located in Great Barrington, Massachusetts. The Institute kindly offered to help with the video recording, providing a location, equipment, and a camera man pro bono.

Introduction
The Great Barrington Declaration – As infectious disease epidemiologists and public health scientists we have grave concerns about the damaging physical and mental health impacts of the prevailing COVID-19 policies and recommend an approach we call Focused Protection.

Coming from both the left and right, and around the world, we have devoted our careers to protecting people. Current lockdown policies are producing devastating effects on short and long-term public health. The results (to name a few) include lower childhood vaccination rates, worsening cardiovascular disease outcomes, fewer cancer screenings and deteriorating mental health – leading to greater excess mortality in years to come, with the working class and younger members of society carrying the heaviest burden. Keeping students out of school is a grave injustice.

The declaration has almost 1M signatures worldwide at the time of writing.

For the entire declaration refer to the link below:

Ref: https://gbdeclaration.org/

WHO World Health Organisation contrived "Pandemic"

Furthermore, as is now well-evidenced, for example by former WHO employee, Astrid Stuckelberger, Grand Jury witness, this "Covid" event never satisfied the criteria for a pandemic. The World Health Organization changed the criteria to **make this a pandemic**. To qualify for a pandemic status the virus must have a high mortality rate for the vast majority of people, which it did never did (with a 99.98% survival rate), and it must have **no known existing treatments—which this "VIRUS" HAD** — in fact, a growing number of very successful treatments. These treatments were banned by the so called "Health" authorities world-wide.

Ref: Appendix I p40 – PDF Download File

It is patently clear from this brief introduction that all was, and still is, not right in the world of "Covid19".

Contrary to all established good medical practices Governments, Health Ministers, Drug and Medicine Authorities, Health Authorities right down to local doctors and the Mainstream Media were in a global lockstep of pushing a false narrative. All the way down to the evil of injecting children who were at zero, we repeat zero, risk from "Covid19".

WHY?

The answers are in the following chapters.

CHAPTER B

WHY A LETTER, A 67 PAGE REPORT WITH 36 APPENDICES, REFUTING THE MAINSTREAM "SARS-COV2/COVID19" NARRATIVE, SENT TO 18 UK GOVERNMENT AUTHORITIES AND MAINSTREAM MEDIA OUTLETS THREE TIMES OVER A SIX-MONTH PERIOD, RECEIVED NOT ONE REPLY

The short answer can only be that the 18 recipients of the letter, Report and Appendices **could not challenge the contents**. If you cannot challenge such documents; the simplest, though not necessarily the best solution, is to ignore it and hope that it will go away. **This matter will never go away**. It is a massive global blood stain on all of our Histories. Let's investigate some of the details:

The persons listed: Boris Johnson, Matt Hancock et al Appendix I p1 et al – PDF Download File were sent **the challenge to refute and rebut the allegations** of two Nobel Prize winners – one the inventor of the PCR Test in 1987/1988, the other the discoverer of HIV, a Nobel prize nominee – the inventor of a working remedy for "Covid19" using a combination of hydroxychloroquine, azithromycin, and zinc which was banned by the governments, medical authorities and the mass media; the architect of mRNA methodologies now personally banned from 'Twitter', Robert F Kennedy – ex-president John F Kennedy's nephew - a 'Big Pharma' trial lawyer, Prof. John Ioannidis, Professor of Medicine (Stanford Prevention Research), of Epidemiology and Population Health, Stanford University USA – the most widely cited expert person in the world in this field and Dr Reiner Fuellmich anti-corporate corruption trial lawyer and many other scientists and lawyers world-wide. These persons and others made these very serious allegations below (and many others):

1. **Dr. Kary Mullis, Nobel Prize winner, inventor of the PCR Test** in/around 1987/1988 quote:

   'It* [PCR test] *does not tell you if you are sick'

   Ref: 13c Report Appendix I p62 [It is not a diagnostic tool for anything!]

2. **'The only way to end the pandemic is universal vaccination.'**

   'Those who pushed this line of argument* [above] *and enabled the gene-based agents* ["vaccines"] *to be injected needlessly into billions of innocent people are guilty of crimes against humanity.' Dr Mike Yeadon author of 'The Covid Lies'

   Ref: 'The Covid Lies' Appendix I p13 et al– PDF Download File

3. **Luc Montagnier, Nobel laureate in medicine for discovering HIV:** quote:

   ***'These "vaccines" are poisons. They are not real vaccines.** As a doctor I knew 21 people who received 2 doses of Pfizer vaccine, there is another person who received Moderna. The 21 died of Creutzfeldt-Jakob disease caused by prions. The 3 vaccines Pfizer, AstraZeneca, Moderna contain a sequence identified by Information Technology as transformation into a prion. There is therefore a known risk to human health.'*

   Ref: https://www.soulask.com/luc-montagnier-they-are-not-vaccines-they-are-poisons-speech-to-the-luxembourg-parliament/

4. **N. Ana Garner, Attorney at Law, USA:** quote: ***'The basis of the [Covid19] pandemic was a big lie...a criminal collaboration…irrefutable evidence of fraud and malfeasance…'***

   Ref: Appendix I p23 – PDF Download File

5. **Dr Zelenko, Nobel Prize nominee** regarding Covid19/"vaccination" procedures quote: ***'Crimes against Humanity' and '1st Degree Murder'***

   https://www.redvoicemedia.com/video/2021/12/dr-zelenko-cuts-through-the-omicron-con-of-fauci-pfizer-the-biden-regimes-global-psychosis-agenda-video/?utm_source=daily-email-breaking&utm_medium=email

6. **Dr Robert Malone,** The architect of mRNA technologies and RNA as a drug, states at the International Covid Summit.

   Quote: ***'In USA FDA* [Food and Drug Administration] *and CDC* [Centres for Disease Control and Prevention] *are acting beyond the law, 'Covid-19' originated in a laboratory using GAIN of FUNCTION technology,* [the] *"vaccinated" are at the highest risk from covid spreading, in Israel* [the] *"vaccinated" are getting infected - they then go to hospital and DIE, the SOCIAL CONTRACT will be destroyed'***

   Ref: https://www.youtube.com/watch?v=EWWvk2SaMS4

   Note: Gain of Function in a "vaccine" in this context, is the result of genetically engineering the "vaccine" to be more lethal, more virulent and more infectious, and mutate or adapt more readily. **Ergo the "vaccines" are de facto Bioweapons/ Chemical Weapons!**

7. **Robert F Kennedy Jr**: Quote:

   'This is a designed human tragedy of Biblical proportions.'

   Ref: Appendix I – PDF Download File p39, Ref 32a page 55

8. **Prof. Michel Chussodovsky - Professor of Economics** quote:

   'Covid19 'pandemic'* [is the] *most serious social-economic crisis in History…'
   'Based on false statistics, 193 countries ordered to close down their economies...'

'the [Covid19] 'pandemic' is economic warfare...' '[Pfizer] "vaccines" programmes were homicide up to 28*th *February 2022, after that date, [Pfizer] had their data and therefore their "vaccines" programmes became murder..."

Ref: Appendix I – PDF Download File Appendix 28 page 75

9. **Dr Reiner Fuellmich Anti-corruption trial lawyer** – quote:

'New evidence from USA Government "vaccine" Adverse Event Reporting System 'VAERS' data, shows that Big Pharma is coordinating between their companies, on a rationalised premeditated deliberate basis, the distribution of toxic [Covid19] "vaccines" that main and kill people.'

Ref: https://www.bitchute.com/video/M0vmjVc5mkQM/

These verbatim quotations are a very small, randomly selected sample from the very many such quotes in the letter, Report and Appendices as explained below:

A letter, a 56-page Report with 4 Appendices the latest version is in Appendix I – PDF Download File - Letter, Report and Appendices were sent to the 18 persons listed below on 15th June 2022 by Royal Mail print copy and by email, requesting refutations and rebuttals of all the allegations by 29th July 2022. **There was Not ONE REPLY from ANYONE.**

A similar letter, an enlarged 66-page Report with 35 Appendices was sent to the same list plus copies to Lord Sumption, and Baroness Harding on 2nd August 2022 by email, under the Freedom of Information Act 2000 (FOI) requesting documentation that presented refutations and rebuttals of all the allegations by 30th September 2022. **There was Not ONE REPLY from ANYONE.**

A similar letter, a further enlarged 67-page Report with 37 Appendices was sent to the same list plus copies to Lord Sumption, and Baroness Harding on 12th October 2022 by email, under the Freedom of Information Act 2000 (FOI) requesting documentation that presented refutations and rebuttals of all the allegations by 30th November 2022. **There was Not ONE REPLY from ANYONE.**

The List of Recipients of The Letter, Report and Appendices

Recipients	**UK Office at the Time c. 2019-2022**
Boris Johnson	**Prime Minister**
Matt Hancock	**Health & Social Care**
Nadhim Zahawi	**"Covid" "Vaccine" Deployment**
Michael Gove	**Cabinet Office**
Sajid Javid	**Health & Social Care**
Suella Braverman	**Attorney General**
Priti Patel	**Home Office**
Baroness Hallett	**Chair Covid Inquiry 2021-**
Christopher Whitty	**Chief Medical Officer/Chief Medical Advisor**

Patrick Vallance	**Chief Scientific Advisor**
June Munro Raine	**CEO MHRA -** Medicines and Healthcare Products Regulatory Agency
Charlie Massey	**CEO GMC –** General Medical Council
Amanda Pritchard	**CEO NHS –** National Health Service
Neil Ferguson	**Researcher** - Imperial College, London
John Witherow	**'The Times'** - Editor
Chris Evans	**'The Telegraph'** - Editor
Katharine Viner	**'The Guardian'** - Editor
Ian Hislop	**'Private Eye'** - Editor

CORONA ACCOUNTABILITY (Covid19) 2022 can only deduce, as the reader may, the reason why there were no rebuttals or refutations to such serious allegations. Those very serious allegations from some of the world's finest minds in this field included – as above:

'Crimes against humanity',

'These "vaccines" are poisons. They are not real vaccines',

'The basis of the* [Covid19] *pandemic was a big lie...a criminal collaboration…irrefutable evidence of fraud and malfeasance…'

'Crimes against Humanity' and 1st Degree Murder'

'Covid-19' originated in a laboratory using GAIN of FUNCTION technology,* [the] *"vaccinated" are at the highest risk from covid spreading, in Israel* [the] *"vaccinated" are getting infected - they then go to hospital and DIE,'

'This is a <u>designed</u> human tragedy of Biblical proportions.'

'Big Pharma is coordinating between their companies, on a rationalised premeditated deliberate basis, the distribution of toxic* [Covid19] *"vaccines" that main and kill people.'

The short answer, as stated above, can only be that **<u>the 18 recipients of the letter, Report and Appendices could not challenge the contents</u>**. If you cannot challenge such a document; the simplest, though not necessarily the best solution, is to ignore it and hope that it will go away. This matter will never go away. This state of affairs, when you consider that it is **unlawful to not reply to a Freedom of Information Request FOIA 2000 within 20 working days** (at a maximum), then the persons/offices not replying are making themselves open not only to ridicule, but to prosecution.

It is rather like a murderer who refuses to give a statement to the Police, refuses to take the stand in a Criminal Court to provide evidence, to obtain his/her fair justice, for fear that the truth will be revealed, and a suitable custodial term will be delivered by the Judge.

This will never go away. There is nowhere for these people to hide. Perhaps they know this.

The reader will find the complete reasons and explanations in the following chapters 1 to 14 and chapter 18.

CHAPTER 1

CONFIDENCE TRICK 1: "SARS-COV2" WAS A NATURAL VIRUS - IT WAS NOT

'The most dangerous bioweapon ever released on the population is "Sars-Cov2"'

Dr Michael McDowell

Ref: https://rumble.com/embed/vonrmq/

It is not being stated that there was **NOT** something or another that caused some form of infection or another world-wide from late 2019 onwards to the present date – November 2022. There was certainly something that appeared to be very virulent and had very debilitating symptoms.

What is being stated is that whatever it was, it was NOT a natural virus.

A generic definition of a virus:

'A virus is a chain of nucleic acids (DNA or RNA) which lives in a host cell uses parts of the cellular machinery to reproduce and releases the replicated nucleic acid chains to infect more cells. A virus is often housed in a protein coat or protein envelope, a protective covering which allows the virus to survive between hosts.'

Ref: https://biologydictionary.net/virus/

In no part of this definition is there any mention of the existence of **human immunodeficiency virus [HIV] within a generic virus.** This is hardly surprising! See Dr Wagh's findings below:

Dr Poornima Wagh, Researcher, 2 PhDs in Virology and Immunology, Santa Barbara, CA, USA

Quote:

***'How do you find HIV* [human immunodeficiency virus] *spike proteins in a 'NOVEL' virus genome? You don't, it's called <u>FRAUD</u>'* [What has been called, by the World Health Organisation 'WHO' etc. "Sars-Cov2" <u>IS NOT</u> a virus!]**

Ref: https://www.bitchute.com/video/btuJXs0glmla/

Ref: Item 2 in letter to Boris Johnson et al Appendix I – p2 PDF Download File

Dr Michael McDowell quoting Dr Francis Boyle a Bioweapon and Law Expert who framed the USA Anti-terrorism ACT

Quotes:

'Sars-Cov2 is an offensive biological war agent made in a lab and engineered with gain of function properties.'

'Sars-Cov2 is a tripartite chimera composed of:

1. ***Sars "virus"***
2. ***Enhanced gain of function properties***
3. ***Genetically combined with HIV'*** **[human immunodeficiency virus]**

'Wuhan Corona genetic analysis provides a gain of function of the 2019 "novel" "coronavirus" for efficient spreading in the human population.'

Gain of function definition: Genetically engineered to be more lethal, more virulent and more infectious, and mutate or adapt more readily.

'The most dangerous bioweapon ever released on the population is "Sars- Cov2"'

Ref: https://rumble.com/embed/vonrmq/

The "Sar-Cov2" "virus" was not an evolutionary virus that we might find in nature, in our natural world. It was engineered by human beings in research labs most probably in USA, perhaps Fort Detrick and Wuhan, China. Some of the funding coming from USA.

Dr Christian Anderson, researcher, in a secret email, some such emails were discussed at a Senate Hearing in USA – January 2022, sent to Dr Fauci, Chief Medical Advisor to the President of United States, the email stated:

'The unusual features of the "Sars-cov2 virus" make up a really small part of the genome so someone has to look really closely at the sequence to see that ***some features look engineered****. Further, I should mention that after discussions Eddy, Bob and Mike* [fellow researchers], *we all find the* ***genome inconsistent with expectations for evolutionary theory****.'*

Dr Charles Leiber, Chair of Harvard University's Chemistry and Chemical Biology Department was involved in bio-weapon technologies at the lab in Wuhan, China which is indicative of USA-China collaboration in engineering the "SarsCov2" "virus" bioweapon.

"Sars-Cov2" has never been isolated

"Sars-Cov2" "virus" has **never been isolated anywhere in the world** and therefore it **DOES NOT EXIST as a scientifically proven, existent "virus"**. Since "Sars-Cov2" has never been isolated according to the established methodologies that have existed for centuries, then it cannot be said to exist from a scientific, medical, virological or indeed any existential standpoint. The reasons why "Sars-Cov2" was never isolated is because such isolation is of no interest to the persons orchestrating their global plan – the Evil300. It was not necessary to isolate the "virus" by such persons because they already knew what it was. Their greater interest is the "vaccines". "Sars-Cov2" and its ensuing illness "Covid19" were simply, primarily instruments of mass fear. Upon this global mass fear, the 'globalists' could oblige upon the global population, mass "vaccination" of experimental drugs that were not only NOT true vaccines but were also NOT trialled nor approved and hence were simply experimental.

As quoted above:

Dr Poornima Wagh, Researcher, 2 PhDs in Virology and Immunology, Santa Barbara, CA, USA

Quote:

'How do you find HIV **[human immunodeficiency virus]** ***spike proteins in a 'NOVEL' virus genome? You don't, it's called FRAUD'*** **[What has been called, by the World Health Organisation 'WHO' etc. "Sars-Cov2" IS NOT a virus!]**

Ref: Item 2 in letter to Boris Johnson et al Appendix I – p5 PDF Download File

Dr Wagh further states:

'Studies of true isolation **[Koch Postulates]** ***from April to September 2020 using tests repeated three times with 1,500 samples resulted in only debris being found! NO "Sars-Cov2/Covid19" or any other virus was found' 'Studies repeated in 7 Universities with the same results'***

The samples failed the **Koch Postulates Examination. Viruses exist in nature, if no virus was found, then the so-called "virus" does not exist in nature and therefore it must be something man-made.** If man-made then it is a **Bioweapon/Chemical Weapon** because of the use of gain of function and the physical harm it has caused and the harm it caused by lockdowns, masks, social distancing in physical and economic terms and its deliberate use between 2019-2022 is indicative of **Mass Murder** and **Genocide**.

Koch Postulates methodology involves taking samples from patients infected with a virus, isolating that virus from all other genetic matter then injecting the isolated virus into known trial subjects. The process is then repeated by taking samples from the deliberately infected trial subjects, isolating the virus and then injecting the virus into other known subjects. To pass the Koch Postulates Test then all injected subjects, in the chain described above, must show EXACTLY the SAME symptoms. If they do, then the isolated material IS a virus, if they do not, then the isolated material is not a virus.

As Dr Wagh states above, in her **tests** ***'...from April to September 2020 using tests repeated three times with 1,500 samples resulted in only debris being found! NO "Sars-Cov2/Covid19" or any other virus was found'***

When undertaking her studies, Dr Wagh and her research staff were in communication with the USA Centers for Disease Control and Prevention 'CDC' and established an on-going relationship and discussions. Dr Wagh asked Robert Redfield, CDC Director, USA if he could assist her team's studies by providing samples. Robert Redfield could not provide samples to Dr Poornima Wagh and her researchers for testing in the laboratories and told the researchers to **call whatever they found "Sars-Cov-2"**!! Robert Redfield in giving this instruction was clearly acting, if not unlawfully, then certainly not within professional and ethical guidelines. The researchers refused; the laboratory was afterwards raided by the Federal Bureau of Investigation FBI (USA) in April 2021. **Computers and paperwork were removed by the FBI!** If this is the behaviour of persons concerned with truth and health care, then we are all lost! This study by Dr Wagh is understood to be the only study of its kind in the world.

Ref: Appendix I – p6 PDF Download File

"Sars-Cov2" - No Records of Isolation Found Anywhere in the World

Furthermore, it has been reported that circa 203 requests all over the world (and rising) for scientific study results for "Sars-Cov-2" **isolation/purification** has resulted in **zero claims** of such isolation/purification. The countries totalled over 30 and included: Australia, Canada, New Zealand, UK, USA, South Africa, Norway, Portugal, Italy, India, etc. **All reported *"No Record Found"*** **[of true "Sars-Cov-2" isolation/purification see Dr Wagh above]**

"Freedom of Information Requests 'FOIs' reveal that health/science institutions around the world (203 and counting!) have no record of SARS-COV-2 isolation/purification, anywhere, ever"

This report states: ***'Would a sane person mix a patient sample (containing various sources of genetic material and never proven to contain any alleged "virus") with transfected monkey kidney cells, fetal bovine serum and toxic drugs, then claim that the resulting concoction is "SARS-COV-2 isolate" and ship it off internationally for use in critical research (including vaccine and test development)?'*** This is a very damning indictment!

Ref: Letter to Boris Johnson et al Appendix I – p1 onwards PDF Download File

Ref: For more details see Christine Massey: christinem@fluoridefreepeel.ca

CHAPTER 2

CONFIDENCE TRICK 2: "SARS-COV2" NATURAL "VIRUS" EXISTED –IT DID NOT

Dr Poornima Wagh, Researcher, 2 PhDs in Virology and Immunology, Santa Barbara, CA, USA

Quote:

"Studies of true isolation **[of the "virus" using Koch Postulates]** ***from April to September 2020 using tests repeated three times with 1,500 samples <u>resulted in only debris being found</u>! <u>NO "Sars-Cov2/Covid19" or any other virus was found"</u> "Studies repeated in 7 Universities – same results"***

Ref: Item 2 in letter to Boris Johnson et al Appendix I – p2 onwards PDF Download File

This study information from Dr Wagh is fully supported by video evidence below from a person who sent a Freedom of Information request to the Government Health & Safety Executive 'HSE' in Ireland. The response formal response by the 'HSE' was that they could not provide documented data that supported the notion that **"Sars Cov2/Covid19"** had at any time been scientifically isolated. Also explained in the previous chapter.

'Ireland's HSE Fails to Produce Evidence for "Sars-Cov2"' – Jan 2021

'This important post serves to spread this information to as wide an audience as possible. Ireland's Ministry of Health responded to a Freedom of Information Request 'FOI' request, saying they could NOT find ANY data in evidence that a "SARS-COV-2" virus had been isolated in laboratory conditions using the scientific method.'

'In effect, the organisation has admitted they have ***no proof the virus exists****, and thus the foundation of lockdowns, social distancing, mask wearing, and most importantly – "VACCINES" - have no basis in science of any kind.'*

Ref: https://rumble.com/vcdxw7-irelands-hse-fails-to-produce-evidence-for-sars-cov-2.html

It has been reported that circa 200 requests all over the world for scientific study results for "Sars-Cov-2" **isolation/purification** has resulted in **<u>zero claims</u>** of such isolation/ purification. The countries included: Australia, Canada, New Zealand, UK, USA, South Africa, Norway, Portugal, Italy, India, etc. **<u>All reported *"No Record Found"*</u> [of "Sars-Cov-2" isolation/purification]**

"Freedom of Information Requests 'FOIs' reveal that health/science institutions around the world (203 and counting!) have no record of SARS-COV-2 isolation/purification, anywhere, ever".

Ref: https://www.fluoridefreepeel.ca/fois-reveal-that-health-science-institutions-around-the-world-have-no-record-of-sars-cov-2-isolation-purification/

Boris Johnson et al were requested **three times** in three separate letters, Report and its Appendices to rebut the allegation that "SarsCov2/Covid19" had never been isolated and therefore did not exist. The second letter stated, 'This is a formal request made both under the Freedom of Information Act 2000 and not under the Freedom of Information Act 2000.' The third letter was sent under The Freedom of Information Act 2000.

There were NO replies.

Ref: Letter, Report/Appendices Appendix I – PDF Download File

Proof the SARS-COV-2 virus does not exist worldwide FOI requests Posted 15 July 2021

Ref: https://forlifeonearth.weebly.com/proof-the-sars-cov-2-virus-does-not-exist.html

We have the evidence that pure, isolated samples of the Covid-19 coronavirus do not exist: a Japanese source has provided us with responses to Freedom of Information requests showing that 10 countries, plus Pfizer itself, do not hold an isolate of SARS-COV-2 (see below).

Thus, the "virus" does not exist in physical reality; it "exists" <u>only in a computer program</u>.

For an example, let's look at the paper entitled:
"Severe Acute Respiratory Syndrome Coronavirus 2 from Patient with Coronavirus Disease, United States" by Harcourt et al. on the Centers for Disease Control and Prevention (CDC) website.

Under the heading "Whole Genome Sequencing," the authors say:

"We designed 37 pairs of nested PCRs spanning the genome on the basis of the coronavirus reference sequence (GenBank accession no. NC045512)."

Critiquing the USA Centers for Disease Control and Prevention 'CDC' paper above, Dr. Tom Cowan says:

'To me, this computer-generation step constitutes scientific fraud.'

'Here is an equivalency: A group of researchers claim to have found a unicorn because they found a piece of a hoof, a hair from a tail, and a snippet of a horn. They then add that information into a computer and program it to re-create the unicorn, and they then claim this computer re-creation is the real unicorn.'

From Ref above:

<u>Pfizer</u> Quotes:
[From an email exchange with a Pfizer customer-service representative]

'The* [Pfizer] *DNA template used does not come from an isolated virus from an infected person.'

'The DNA template (Sars-Cov, Gen Bank MN9089473) was generated via a combination of gene synthesis and recombinant DNA technology.'

The total madness of this situation becomes clear when one analysis the responsibilities of those responsible.

How are we meant to believe, that Pfizer, Moderna, Johnson & Johnson and AstraZeneca, the companies who are supposedly offering the world safe "vaccines" **against** "Sars-Cov2" have not isolated the offending "virus". It is not unreasonable to assume that they would be very keen and the first organisations to do so, so that they can quickly and efficiently design the appropriate "vaccines" to solve the cause of the "Covid19" illness!

However, NONE of these companies have isolated the "Sars-Cov2" virus. Since we are approaching 3 years after the Wuhan, China first outbreak in December 2019, then one may reasonably assume that the companies, responsible for the world's health in this regard - Pfizer, Moderna, Johnson & Johnson and AstraZeneca, have absolutely NO intention of doing so despite the fact that it is their primary responsibility. If that is not an admission of GUILT, what is?

It is important to note here, that the isolation of the "virus" should have occurred prior to the design and creation use of vaccines so that the "vaccines" could have been appropriately designed based on the inherent nature of the "virus" that the isolation would have revealed! This DID NOT happen!

They have no need to isolate the "virus" to find out its true constituents because their associates made it! Consequently, presumably they already know that it contains HIV spike proteins. Refer to the results of Dr Poornima Wagh's research below, referenced also in other chapters.

Dr Poornima Wagh, Researcher, 2 PhDs in Virology and Immunology, Santa Barbara, CA, USA

Quote:

***'How do you find HIV* [human immunodeficiency virus] *spike proteins in a 'NOVEL' virus genome? You don't, it's called FRAUD'* [What has been called, by the World Health Organisation 'WHO' etc. "Sars-Cov2" IS NOT a virus!]**

From the same reference URL above, regarding UK Authorities; the UK Government Office for Science on 20th August 2020 and on 19th March 2021 stated that they could not provide documents supporting that the isolation of 'Sas-Cov2' had occurred. Further, the UK Health and Safety Executive on 3rd November 2020 stated that they could not provide documents supporting that the isolation of 'Sas-Cov2' had occurred.

China's Top 'CDC' epidemiologist confirmed that China has never isolated the Covid-19 "Virus". 23.1.2021

Dr Wuzunyou Chinese Centre for Disease Control quote:

'They didn't isolate the virus.'

Furthermore, the UK General Medical Council GMC, the UK National Health Service NHS, Nadhim Zahawi Office of "Covid" "Vaccine" Deployment, **could NOT provide proof of the isolation and therefore existence of "SarsCov2" nor the safety of the "vaccines"!! Proofs requested:**

1. Proof of the existence of the SARS-CoV-2 virus by research describing the isolation of the SARS-CoV-2 virus aka COVID-19 in human beings, by scientific analysis of samples taken directly from a diseased patient, where the patient samples were not first combined with any other source of genetic material. Note: The word "isolate" means: a thing (SARS-CoV-2/COVID-19) is separated from all other material surrounding it. I am not requesting information where so-called "isolation" of SARS-CoV-2 refers to: - the culturing of something, or - the performance of an amplification test (PCR), or - the sequencing of something. The research study methodology may require the use of Koch Postulates.
2. Proof that all the vaccines approved for use in UK such as: Moderna vaccine, Oxford/AstraZeneca vaccine, Pfizer/BioNTech vaccine and any other vaccine approved for use in UK but not here listed, are all safe for human use and do not contain any graphene oxide or any other substances in any way harmful to humans.

See Appendix II p 196

'Busted: 11 COVID Assumptions Based on Fear Not Fact' – 13th July 2020

Ref: https://www.globalresearch.ca/11-covid-assumptions-based-fear-not-fact/5718352

'COVID assumptions – the assumptions people make about COVID, how dangerous it is, how it spreads and what we need to do to stop it – are running rampant, running far more wildly than the supposed virus SARS-CoV2 itself. The coldly calculated campaign of propaganda surrounding this 'pandemic' has achieved its aim. Besieged with a slew of contradictory information coming from all angles, people in general have succumbed to confusion. Some have given up trying to understand the situation and found it is just easier to obey official directives, even if it means giving up long-held rights. Below is a list of commonly held COVID assumptions which, if you believe them, will make you much more likely to submit to the robotic, insane and abnormal conditions of the **New Normal** *– screening, testing, contact tracing, monitoring, surveillance, mask-wearing, social distancing, quarantine, and isolation, with mandatory vaccination and microchipping to come.'*

'As covered in previous articles, the PCR test (Polymerase Chain Reaction) was invented by scientist **Kary Mullis** as a manufacturing technique (since it is able to replicate DNA sequences millions and billions of times), not as a diagnostic tool.

COVID or SARS-CoV2 fails Koch's postulates - see Chapter 1.

The virus which shut the world down has still to this day never been isolated, purified, and re-injected, or in other words, has never been 100% proven to exist, nor 100% proven to be the cause of the disease.'

CHAPTER 3

CONFIDENCE TRICK 3: "SARS-COV2/COVID19" WAS HIGH RISK – IT WAS NOT

Dr Reiner Fuellmich - Anti-Corporate Corruption Lawyer, Founder 'International Crime Investigative Committee' 'ICIC'

Quote:

'"Covid-19" "virus" is no more dangerous than the common flu! Typically 0.14%-0.15% fatality of population.'

Ref: https://rumble.com/vmvlnv-international-lawyer-dr-reiner-fuellmich-speaks-out.html

John P. A. Ioannidis - Physician Scientist Stanford University USA – most cited expert in the world in this field.

Quote:

'Acknowledging residual uncertainties, the available evidence suggests average global IFR **[Infection Fatality Ratio]** ***of ~0.15%'***

Ref: 2b Appendix I – p58 PDF Download File

The figure of 0.15% is the same as that pronounced by Dr Reiner Fuellmich above and quoted elsewhere in the Report Appendix I – Appendix 27 p75 PDF Download File

The inflated risk was based on ***computer models*** (rubbish data in, must result in, rubbish results out) designed by Imperial College's (London UK) **Neil Ferguson** that were proven to be completely divorced from any form of reality – just as his previous models for swine flu were too. These models predicted tens of million deaths in a pandemic that was compared to the Spanish flu, **the deadliest epidemic in modern times**. The only option, warned the report, would be radical physical distancing of the entire population, potentially for 18 months, until a vaccine was available. It appears that Neil Ferguson was not aware that the typical time to market of a new "vaccine" is 6 to 10 years minimum, rather longer than 18 months!

Ref: ***'The Flawed Covid19 Model that Locked Down Canada'***

Ref: https://www.iedm.org/wp-content/uploads/2020/06/note032020_en.pdf

In other words, his completely inaccurate computer models predicted an estimated "infection fatality rate" (IFR) of 3% (for comparison, seasonal influenza (flu) is generally considered to have a typical IFR of 0.1%-0.14%). This means it cannot be argued that the risk of Covid19 is significantly different or more dangerous than that from some seasonal influenza epidemics. There are many reports that people supposedly dying from Covid19, died with secondary symptoms (***co-morbidities i.e., underlying conditions)*** that were a hugely significant contribution to the cause of the death. However, the "cause" of death was dubiously recorded as Covid19. Presumably to increase the fear factor to increase "vaccine" uptake. It was widely reported that the number of deaths **FROM** Covid19 were highly inflated for financial gain. If a person had tested positive from the **nonsense PCR Test** (see below) within 28 days of death, the death was recorded as 'with Covid19' or 'Covid19' was entered on the death certificate, despite underlying health issues that were the true, inherent cause of death. There were bizarre reports of people dying from road traffic accidents (dripping in blood with bodies full of broken bones) and at the 'hospital' their death was reported as 'Covid19'.

Ref: https://www.cnsnews.com/article/washington/melanie-arter/cdc-director-i-think-youre-correct-about-inflated-covid-death

The risk of Covid19 was purposely inflated by use of inappropriate PCR tests

The World Health Organisation WHO needed "cases" in order to declare a Public Health Emergency of International Concern 'PHEIC', employed a never before used **Drosten-PCR test**. Yet, contagion can never be detected by PCR because the test has very high incidences of false-positives.

Ref: The Grand Jury Day 3 February 13 2022 URL link: https://odysee.com/@GrandJury:f/Grand-Jury-Day-3-en-online:7 hrs:mins:sec 01:51:46 to 02:09:20, Dr. Sona Pekova, Molecular Biologist, Czech Republic ***and*** hrs:min:sec 01:11:00 to 01:17:48, Prof. Dr. Ulrike Kammerer, Virologist & Immunologist, Germany

This is because the test is run on cycle thresholds (CTs) (Amplifications) and for Covd19 they were run at well above the **recommended rate 25 CTs maximum** (in the **UK NHS run at over 40 CTs (false "science")** versus 25 recommended **maximum**) and using three markers in the body (subsequently reduced to two) were used to falsely give an impression of 'rising covid19 infections' to the public.

Ref: The Grand Jury Day 3 February 13 2022 URL link: https://odysee.com/@GrandJury:f/Grand-Jury-Day-3-en-online:7 Dr. Astrid Stuckelberger, International Health Scientist and Researcher, Switzerland min:secs 8:10 to 15:20

In order for a test to truly detect "SARS Cov-2" many different assays needed to be able to catch all the individual strains of virus. However Drosten designed PCR in a complicated way, so as to make it applicable to anything therefore creating many false positives. The task was not to make a PCR test that was specific, but a test to produce "case" numbers.

Ref: The Grand Jury Day 3 February 13 2022 URL link: https://odysee.com/@GrandJury:f/Grand-Jury-Day-3-en-online:7

Dr. Astrid Stuckelberger, International Health Scientist and Researcher, Switzerland min:secs 8:10 to 15:20

Covid *deaths* were over-counted worldwide based on the PCR test

We are lead to believe that "millions" have died '*of* Covid' – millions worldwide die every year. Yet all Covid deaths, anywhere, are based "on a test within 28 days of a positive (PCR) test". Whilst the average age of "Covid" death – *with co-morbidities i.e., underlying conditions* – was 84 years (deaths after the roll-out of the "jabs" cannot be divorced from the effects of the "jabs") the average age of death in normal times is 82.5 years i.e. the majority of those dying of Covid were/are *older* than the average age of natural death!

'In the midst of everything COVID, people were ... putting down that cause of death as COVID ... It is important to go back and do this accounting to see if COVID was actually the cause of death.'

Ref: https://www.westernjournal.com/right-experts-confirm-covid-deaths-massively-inflated-actual-numbers-dramatically-lower-official-count/

'It is likely that the cumulative COVID-19 deaths in countries like USA, UK, and Spain and other similar high-income countries have been overestimated. Some of this over-estimation has slowly started to be gradually recognized as of this writing, e.g., in June and July 2021, Alameda and Santa Clara counties in California have reduced their COVID-19 deaths by 25% and 22%, respectively, trying to address over counting.'

'Excess deaths should be ***scrutinized for death causes accentuated by the "pandemic"*** *versus by measures taken against the pandemic, e.g., deaths due to disruption of health care, opioid overdoses, suicides, diseases of despair, starvation, tuberculosis, and more.'*

'Autopsies also find many more problems than are otherwise reported. However, autopsies are exceedingly rare.'

Quotes: John P A Ioannidis – Stanford University USA

Ref: https://link.springer.com/article/10.1007/s10654-021-00787-9

"Sars-Cov2/Covid19" was NOT high risk

There were treatments for this "virus" available and ready to use immediately!

From the very start of this "worldwide health crisis", there were many prominent scientists and medical doctors who exclaimed how they were successfully treating many thousands of "Covid" patients using existing drugs that are known for their safety and efficacy. There is for example the world-famous French professor Didier Raoult, director of one of the largest research groups in infectious diseases and microbiology. He is the most cited microbiologist in Europe according to ISI and has trained more than 457 foreign scientists in his lab since

1998 with more than 1950 articles referred in ISI or Pubmed and is considered the world's foremost expert on infectious diseases. **Professor Raoult started treating "Covid" patients with a medicine that has been around for over sixty years and is famous for its safety and efficiency in defeating coronaviruses: hydroxychloroquine.**

Professor Raoult treated over four thousand patients with hydroxychloroquine + azithromycin and virtually all of them recovered, except for a handful of very elderly who already had several morbidities.

This incredible success inspired many other medical doctors around the world to start using the same drug. In The Netherlands, **Dr. Rob Elens gave all his covid patients hydroxychloroquine combined with zinc and saw a 100% recovery rate in an average of four days.** Nobody needed to be hospitalized. Along with 2,700+ other medical professionals, this physician sent a letter to the Dutch government, asking them to include HCQ into the standard protocol. Dr. Elens and other Dutch medical doctors set up a 'COVID-19 Self Care' website, with information on how to prevent and overcome "COVID-19", using HCQ and zinc.

In New York, the family practitioner Dr. Vladimir Zelenko treated over 500 covid patients at the beginning of the pandemic with hydroxychloroquine + zinc + azithromycin. He also had a 100% recovery rate, with hardly any side effects, and no hospitalizations. As of August 2021, **Dr. Zelenko and his team successfully treated over 6,000 "Covid" patients**. He developed a protocol to treat "COVID19" which became world-famous and is saving the lives of millions of people around the world. The Zelenko Protocol is used by for example the online telemedicine platform https://www.speakwithanmd.com/ and the vast network of 800,000+ members of America's Frontline Doctors.

Hundreds of studies confirm the effectiveness of HCQ in treating COVID-19 and preventing hospitalization and death.

World leading scientists Dr. Pierre Kory and Dr. Peter McCullough are both the most published medical experts in their field. Both these physicians and their teams have successfully treated tens of thousands of "Covid" patients using for example **Ivermectin**. Dr. Kory and his team of top medical experts studied the entire medical literature for over nine months and found that Ivermectin proves to be a miracle drug that effectively prevents and treats "COVID-19".

63 peer reviewed studies confirm the effectiveness of Ivermectin in treating "COVID"

Biophysicist Andreas Kalcker used chlorine dioxide to slash the daily death rate of 100 to 0, in Bolivia and was asked to treat the military, police, and politicians in several Latin American nations. His worldwide network 'COMUSAV.com' consists of thousands of physicians, academics, scientists, and lawyers who are promoting this effective treatment.

With several options to successfully treat COVID-19, why is there still such an outcry for a vaccine? **And why is the majority of the population not even aware of the available treatments?** The answer is shocking and shows once more what is going on in our world...

All over the world physicians who were successfully treating "Covid" patients, encountered the unthinkable: they were intimidated and shut down by the government.

America's Frontline Doctors informed the world about the safe and effective cures for "Covid", during their first White Coat Summit in 2020. This broadcast was viewed over twenty million times in a few hours, but then they were shut down all across the board: Facebook, Youtube, Twitter, and even their website was taken down by Squarespace.

It is clear that there was NO "pandemic" and there was NO NEED for the Bio-Weapon/ Chemical Weapon "vaccines". There was no "Covid19" "pandemic" because the fatality figures were no higher than the common flu (0.14%) and there were plenty of already available treatments. However, the fatality rates were deliberately inflated and the available treatments suppressed.

There are perhaps only two terms that are applicable to these activities, in consideration that they were implemented against the interest of the entire world's "democratically free" population of 6Bn people, and they are '**mass murder**' and '**genocide**'.

For more details on these unlawful activities go to Chapters 13 and 18.

CHAPTER 4

CONFIDENCE TRICK 4: "SARS-COV-2/COVID19" WAS A PANDEMIC – IT WAS NOT

Dr Blaylock, visiting professor in the biology department at Belhaven College, USA

Quote:

'the COVID-19 pandemic is one of the most manipulated infectious disease events in history, characterized by official lies in an unending stream lead by government bureaucracies, medical associations, medical boards, the media, and international agencies.'

Ref: Appendix I – PDF Download File Refs: p15, Ref: [3a] p53, Ref: [6a] p53

'We have witnessed a long list of unprecedented intrusions into medical practice, including attacks on medical experts, destruction of medical careers among doctors refusing to participate in killing their patients and a massive regimentation of health care, led by non-qualified individuals with enormous wealth, power and influence.'

Ref: ***'COVID UPDATE: What is the truth?'*** Surg Neurol Int 2022;13:167

Ref: https://www.ncbi.nlm.nih.gov/pmc/articles/PMC9062939/

Dr Reiner Fuellmich et al

'there is and was no coronavirus "pandemic", rather only a long-planned, PCR test "casedemic"'

Ref: ***Grand Jury Proceedings"*** (***Day 1 - Opening Statements*** **mins:secs 19:32 to 37:34**) **URL link:** https://odysee.com/@GrandJury:f/Grand-Jury-1-EN:0

In ***'COVID UPDATE: What is the truth?'*** Surg Neurol Int 2022;13:167 Dr Blaylock

Dr Blaylock makes a thorough and compelling condemnation upon this so called "pandemic" below:

Medical Treatments not Based on Accurate Science
'For the first time in American history a president, governors, mayors, hospital administrators and federal bureaucrats are determining medical treatments based not on accurate scientifically based or even experience based information, but rather to force the acceptance of special forms

of care and "prevention"—including Remdesivir, [a dangerous drug] *use of respirators and ultimately a series of essentially untested messenger RNA "vaccines". For the first time in history medical treatment, protocols are not being formulated based on the experience of the physicians treating the largest number of patients successfully, but rather individuals and bureaucracies that have never treated a single patient—including Anthony Fauci, Bill Gates, EcoHealth Alliance, the CDC, WHO, state public health officers and hospital administrators.'*

Media Manipulation and Control

'The media (TV, newspapers, magazines, etc), medical societies, state medical boards and the owners of social media have appointed themselves to be the sole source of information concerning this so-called "pandemic". Websites have been removed, highly credentialed and experienced clinical doctors and scientific experts in the field of infectious diseases have been demonized, careers have been destroyed and all dissenting information has been labelled "misinformation" and "dangerous lies", even when sourced from top experts in the fields of virology, infectious diseases, pulmonary critical care, and epidemiology. These blackouts of truth occur even when this information is backed by extensive scientific citations from some of the most qualified medical specialists in the world. Incredibly, even individuals, such as Dr. Michael Yeadon, a retired ex-Chief Scientist, and vice-president for the science division of Pfizer Pharmaceutical Company in the UK, who charged the company with making an extremely dangerous "vaccine", is ignored and demonized. ***Further, he, along with other highly qualified scientists have stated that no one should take this "vaccine".*** *'*

True Experts' Advice Ignored and Personally Attacked

'Dr. Peter McCullough, one of the most cited experts in his field, who has successfully treated over 2000 COVID patients by using a protocol of early treatment (which the so-called experts completely ignored), has been the victim of a particularly vicious assault by those benefiting financially from the "vaccines". He has published his results in peer reviewed journals, reporting an 80% reduction in hospitalizations and a 75% reduction in deaths by using early treatment. Despite this, he is under an unrelenting series of attacks by the information controllers, none of which have treated a single patient.'

Medical Authorities Not Offering Early Treatment

'Neither Anthony Fauci, the CDC, WHO nor any medical governmental establishment has ever offered any early treatment other than Tylenol, hydration and call an ambulance once you have difficulty breathing. This is unprecedented in the entire history of medical care as early treatment of infections is critical to saving lives and preventing severe complications. Not only have these medical organizations and federal lapdogs not even suggested early treatment, they attacked anyone who attempted to initiate such treatment with all the weapons at their disposal—loss of license, removal of hospital privileges, shaming, destruction of reputations and even arrest.'

Professional Medical Freedom Denied

'A good example of this outrage against freedom of speech and providing informed consent information is the recent suspension by the medical board in Maine of Dr. Meryl Nass' medical license and the ordering of her to undergo a psychiatric evaluation for prescribing Ivermectin

and sharing her expertise in this field. I know Dr, Nass personally and can vouch for her integrity, brilliance and dedication to truth. Her scientific credentials are impeccable. This behaviour by a medical licensing board is reminiscent of the methodology of the Soviet KGB during the period when dissidents were incarcerated in psychiatric gulags to silence their dissent.'

Ghost-Written Articles Containing Manipulated Data

'Ghost-written articles involve using planning companies whose job it is to design articles containing manipulated data to support a pharmaceutical product and then have these articles accepted by high-impact clinical journals, that is, the journals most likely to affect clinical decision making of doctors. Further, they supply doctors in clinical practice with free reprints of these manipulated articles. The Guardian [UK Newspaper] *found 250 companies engaged in this ghost-writing business. The final step in designing these articles for publication in the most prestigious journals is to recruit well recognized medical experts from prestigious institutions, to add their name to these articles. These recruited medical authors are either paid upon agreeing to add their name to these pre- written articles or they do so for the prestige of having their name on an article in a prestigious medical journal.'*

'Of vital importance is the observation by experts in the field of medical publishing that nothing has been done to stop this abuse. Medical ethicists have lamented that because of this widespread practice "you can't trust anything." While some journals insist on disclosure information, most doctors reading these articles ignore this information or excuse it and several journals make disclosure more difficult by requiring the reader to find the disclosure statements at another location. Many journals do not police such statements and omissions by authors are common and without punishment.'

Big Pharma Controls the Media

'As concerns the information made available to the public, virtually all the media is under the control of these pharmaceutical giants or others who are benefitting from this "pandemic". Their stories are all the same, both in content and even wording. Orchestrated cover-ups occur daily and massive data exposing the lies being generated by these information controllers are hidden from the public. All data coming over the national media (TV, newspaper and magazines), as well as the local news you watch every day, comes only from "official" sources—most of which are lies, distortions or completely manufactured out of whole cloth—all aimed to deceive the public.'

Hospital Administrators Have Totalitarian Control

'While these attacks on free speech are terrifying enough, even worse is the virtually universal control hospital administrators have exercised over the details of medical care in hospitals. These hirelings are now instructing doctors which treatment protocols they will adhere to and which treatments they will not use, no matter how harmful the "approved" treatments are or how beneficial the "unapproved" treatments are.'

'Never in the history of American medicine have hospital administrators dictated to its physicians how they will practice medicine and what medications they can use. The CDC has no authority to dictate to hospitals or doctors concerning medical treatments. Yet, most physicians complied without the slightest resistance.'

Hospital Administrators Have Caused Mass Deaths

'When this "pandemic" started, hospitals were ordered by the CDC to follow a treatment protocol that resulted in the deaths of hundreds of thousands of patients, most of whom would have recovered had proper treatments been allowed. ***The majority of these deaths could have been prevented had doctors been allowed to use early treatment with such products as Ivermectin, hydroxy-chloroquine and a number of other safe drugs and natural compounds****. It has been estimated, based on results by physicians treating the most covid patients successfully, that of the 800,000 people that we are told died from Covid,* ***640,000 could have not only been saved****, but could have, in many cases, returned to their pre-infection health status had mandated early treatment with these proven methods been used.* ***This neglect of early treatment constitutes mass murder.'***

Dr Blaylock is a leading retired USA Neurosurgeon. Neurosurgeons are not typically attuned to hyperbole. His condemnation of the "Covid19" "pandemic" is clear, quietly assertive and fully in tune with similar reports by those physicians and scientist who have the courage to speak the truth.

Let's look again at the exporting and importing of PCR Test Kits:

Let's repeat our simple test:

Type into your browser (Google etc) on your mobile phone, tablet or laptop the following:

382200 export 2017

382200 is the global product code for the PCR Medical Test Kits as defined by WITS (World Bank) World Integrated Trade Solution. The figures state that the top global 5 exporters in 2017 were:

USA exported 6.57US$Bn, EU exported 6.36US$Bn, Germany exported 4.25US$Bn Netherlands US$1.96Bn, UK 1.78US$BN – all in 2017!

Then type in:

382200 import 2017

Scroll down the tables displayed, for both '382200 export 2017' and '382200 import 2017' and you will observe that practically the entire world circa 195 countries were in the business of exporting and importing PCR Medical Test Kits in 2017!!

The first outbreak of "Covid19" was announced by the World Health Organisation 'WHO' on 31st December 2019. Assuming that to have this huge amount of PCR Test Kits available for export in 2017, they would have to be designed/defined in say 2015, then manufactured in 2016. **This would mean that PCR Test Kits were first being conceived in 2015 a full 5 years before the WHO announced the "virus"!! How does that make sense?!**

Here is an explanation:

Representatives from c. 195 countries – the entire world – did not convene in a football stadium or other building suitably sized to accommodate all of them, (all with little designatory country flags to distinguish one from another) and discuss the whys and wherefores of how to globally initiate, specify, design, approve, manufacture, and **export** to every country in the world, internationally recognised and approved PCR Medical Test Kits all commencing at exactly the same time in 2017!

Ref: https://wits.worldbank.org/trade/comtrade/en/country/ALL/year/2017/tradeflow/Exports/partner/WLD/nomen/h5/product/382200

The complexity of the logistics of this enormous global exercise is not to be underestimated. All of these exporters have to produce PCR Test Kits that satisfy the local individual Health and Safety guidelines of all of the individual countries they export to! For this to work and it obviously did, the only way would be that this was NOT organised at the sovereign state national level. This is simply not feasible or believable. This process must have been meticulously planned and organised at a pan-global level, a level of authority that was above that of sovereign national state governments. The only organisations that have that global power and reach are (plus possibly a few others less well known):

United Nations 'UN'
World Bank
World Health Organisation 'WHO'
World Economic Forum 'WEF'

As you are no doubt aware, businesses world-wide use sophisticated market intelligence metrics to ascertain the risk involved in developing and bringing to market a new product. They only bring to market products that pass their stringent risk assessments. How can it possibly be, that the entire world of business agreed, (individually or together) at the same time, that the PCR Medical Test Kits passed their stringent market risk assessment? **The short answer was that no risk assessment was required!** This is possibly the first time in History that such a complex, multifarious, country inter-dependent, global project has taken place without the requirement for any risk assessment whatsoever!

The global power, control and falsely inflicted fear caused the majority of people in UK and the world to receive "vaccines" that had not undergone full clinical trials and that were rushed to market in a matter of a year or so. True vaccines typically take 7 to 10 years to bring to market using rigorous testing and full clinical trials. The Covid19 "vaccines" appeared on the market in a matter of 11 months. The 'WHO' announced the "virus" to the public on 31st December 2019, the UK Government released "vaccines" to the public on 8th December 2020 a total of 11 months later. These vaccines have never undergone full clinical trials so the unsuspecting public allowed Pfizer – the proud Corporation, owner of the largest ever fine for criminal activities for anything in USA (see Ref below) - to inject into their bodies **experimental substances** that they knew nothing of, and therefore did not, and could not, provide **"informed consent"(a legal obligation)** and thereby became an unsuspecting new global 'breed' as part of a "vaccine" experiment. The entire unsuspecting world population was subjected to the **largest human "vaccination" experiment** in the History of the World.

The evidence, yet again, is clear that this was no "pandemic" – it was planned. Who had foreknowledge of what and when did they have it?

Further evidence of foreknowledge is to be found in official correspondence between various US official bodies:

Confidential Documents reveal Moderna sent mRNA Coronavirus Vaccine Candidate to University Researchers weeks before emergence of "Covid" 18th June 2021

A confidentiality agreement shows potential coronavirus vaccine candidates were transferred from Moderna to the University of North Carolina in 2019, nineteen days prior to the emergence of the alleged Covid-19 causing virus in Wuhan, China.

Ref:https://expose-news.com/2021/06/18/confidential-documents-reveal-moderna-sent-mrna-coronavirus-vaccine-candidate-to-university-researchers-weeks-before-emergence-of-covid-19/

The confidentially agreement which can be viewed **here** states that providers 'Moderna' alongside the 'National Institute of Allergy and Infectious Diseases' (NIAID) agreed to transfer 'mRNA coronavirus vaccine candidates' developed and jointly-owned by NIAID and Moderna to recipients 'The University of North Carolina at Chapel Hill' on the 12th December 2019. Refer to the Public Health Service, Material Transfer Agreement that follows.

PUBLIC HEALTH SERVICE

MATERIAL TRANSFER AGREEMENT

This Material Transfer Agreement ("MTA") has been adopted for use by the National Institutes of Health, the Food and Drug Administration and the Centers for Disease Control and Prevention, collectively referred to herein as the Public Health Service ("PHS") in all transfers of research material (Research Material) whether PHS is identified below as its Provider or Recipient.

Providers: *National Institute of Allergy and Infectious Diseases, National Institutes of Health ("NIAID")*
ModernaTX, Inc ("Moderna")

Recipient: The University of North Carolina at Chapel Hill

1. Provider agrees to transfer to Recipient's Investigator the following Research Material:

mRNA coronavirus vaccine candidates developed and jointly-owned by NIAID and Moderna.

Found on page 105 of the agreement

The material transfer agreement was signed the December 12th, 2019, by Ralph Baric, PhD, at the University of North Carolina at Chapel Hill, and then signed by Jacqueline Quay, Director of Licensing and Innovation Support at the University of North Carolina on December 16th, 2019.

The agreement was also signed by two representatives of the NIAID, one of whom was Amy F. Petrik PhD, a technology transfer specialist who signed the agreement on December 12th, 2019, at 8:05 am. The other signatory was Barney Graham MD PhD, an investigator for the NIAID; however, this signature was not dated.

The final signatories on the agreement were Sunny Himansu, Moderna's Investigator, and Shaun Ryan, Moderna's Deputy General Councel. Both signatures were made on December 17th, 2019.

All of these signatures were made prior to any knowledge of the alleged emergence of the novel coronavirus "Sars-Cov2". It wasn't until December 31st, 2019, that the World Health Organisation (WHO) became aware of an alleged cluster of viral pneumonia cases in Wuhan, China. But even at this point they had not determined that an alleged new coronavirus was to blame, instead stating the pneumonia was of "unknown cause".

It was not until January 9th 2020 that the WHO reported Chinese authorities had determined the outbreak was due to a novel coronavirus which later became known as "SARS-CoV-2" with the alleged resultant disease dubbed "COVID-19".

So why was an mRNA coronavirus vaccine candidate developed by Moderna being transferred to the University of North Carolina on December 12th, 2019?

The evidence, yet again, is clear that this was no "pandemic" – it was planned. Who had foreknowledge of what and when did they have it?

The same Moderna that have had an mRNA "coronavirus vaccine" authorised for emergency use only in both the United Kingdom and United States to allegedly combat "Covid-19".

What did Moderna know that we didn't? In 2019 there was not one singular coronavirus posing a threat to humanity which would warrant a vaccine, and evidence suggests there hasn't been a singular coronavirus posing a threat to humanity throughout 2020 and 2021 either. [Nor throughout 2022 – existing treatments being available.]

Considering the fact a faulty PCR test has been used at a **falsely high cycle rate**, hospitals have been empty in comparison to previous years, statistics show just 0.2% of those allegedly infected have died within 28 days of an alleged positive test result, the majority of those deaths by a mile have been people over the age of 85, and a mass of those deaths were caused by a drug called midazolam, which causes respiratory depression, and respiratory arrest.

Ref: **Midazolam Murder Case UK** – Michael O'Bernicia *'...we will lay a new set of charges against 49 [and still counting] defendants during the next week or so,...to have the Midazolam Murders case listed for trial by jury.'* Posted 24th May 2022

[Matt Hancock – UK Cabinet Minister for Health & Social Care is amongst the defendants.]

Ref: https://www.thebernician.net/tgbms-class-action-midazolam-murders-pcp-move-forward/

CHAPTER 5

CONFIDENCE TRICK 5: "COVID19" RESULTED FROM A NATURAL VIRUS – IT DID NOT

Dr Poornima Wagh, Researcher, 2 PhDs in Virology and Immunology, Santa Barbara, CA, USA

Quote:

"Studies of true isolation **[of the "virus" using Koch Postulates]** ***from April to September 2020 using tests repeated three times with 1,500 samples resulted in only debris being found! NO "Sars-Cov2/Covid19" or any other virus was found" "Studies repeated in 7 Universities – same results"***

Ref: Item 2 in letter to Boris Johnson et al Appendix I – p5 PDF Download File

It is absolutely preposterous that Pfizer, Moderna, Johnson & Johnson and AstraZeneca, on the very first reports of the outbreak of the "virus" in December 2019, did not IMMEDIATELY set about truly isolating the "virus" by centrifugal techniques and Koch postulates in their own research laboratories or in research laboratories that they fund. This activity is slap bang at the very beginning of any critical path analysis! It is not possible, to resolve, any problem whatsoever, without first defining the problem. The problem of the "virus" is in the make-up in its molecular composition (found under isolation) and its viral nature was to be found in its response to tests under Koch postulates. Without these proven tests, NOTHING could truly be achieved in trying to deal with the "virus".

Pfizer Quotes:
[From an email exchange with a Pfizer customer-service representative]

'The **[Pfizer]** ***DNA template used does not come from an isolated virus from an infected person.'***

'The DNA template (Sars-Cov, Gen Bank MN9089473) was generated via a combination of gene synthesis and recombinant DNA technology.'

The total madness of this situation becomes clear when one analyses the duty of care of those responsible.

How are we meant to believe, that Pfizer, Moderna, Johnson & Johnson and AstraZeneca, the companies who are supposedly offering the world safe "vaccines" **against** "Sars-Cov2"/ "Covid19" were so negligent to have not isolated the offending "virus". It is not unreasonable to assume that they would be very keen and the first organisations to do so, so that they can quickly and efficiently design the appropriate "vaccines" to solve the cause of the "Covid19" illness! However, judging by the company's track records in USA courts, we have every reason to believe Pfizer, Moderna, Johnson & Johnson and AstraZeneca company's deplorable negligence.

However, NONE of these companies have isolated the "Sars-Cov2" virus. Since we are approaching 3 years after the Wuhan, China first outbreak in December 2019, then one may reasonably assume that the companies, responsible for the world's health in this regard - Pfizer, Moderna, Johnson & Johnson and AstraZeneca, have absolutely NO intention of doing so despite the fact that it is their primary responsibility. If that is not an admission of GUILT, what is?

They have no need to isolate the "virus" to find out its true constituents because their associates made it! Consequently, presumably they already know that it contains HIV spike proteins. Refer to the results of Dr Poornima Wagh's research below, referenced also in other chapters.

Dr Poornima Wagh, Researcher, 2 PhDs in Virology and Immunology, Santa Barbara, CA, USA

Quote:

'How do you find HIV **[human immunodeficiency virus]** ***spike proteins in a 'NOVEL' virus genome? You don't, it's called FRAUD'*** **[What has been called, by the World Health Organisation 'WHO' etc. "Sars-Cov2" IS NOT a virus!]**

Furthermore, worldwide Freedom of Information Act Requests FOIA have not been able to produce proof of the existence of "Sars-Cov2" by truly scientific isolation.

Ref: https://forlifeonearth.weebly.com/proof-the-sars-cov-2-virus-does-not-exist.html

From the same reference URL above, regarding UK Authorities; the UK Government Office for Science on 20th August 2020 and on 19th March 2021 stated that they could not provide documents supporting that the isolation of 'Sas-Cov2' had occurred. Further, the UK Health and Safety Executive on 3rd November 2020 stated that they could not provide documents supporting that the isolation of 'Sas-Cov2' had occurred.

China's Top 'CDC' epidemiologist confirmed that China has never isolated the Covid-19 "Virus". 23.1.2021

Dr Wuzunyou Chinese Centre for Disease Control quote:

'They didn't isolate the virus.' [To isolate a virus is to determine its inherent constituents]

Dr Peter McCullough reveals the "Covid-19" "Vaccines" are Bioweapons, and a CDC Whistle-Blower has confirmed 50,000 Americans have died due to the jabs.
- 24th June 2021

Ref: https://expose-news.com/2021/06/24/dr-peter-mccullough-reveals-the-covid-19-vaccines-are-bioweapons-and-a-cdc-whistle-blower-has-confirmed-50000-americans-have-died-due-to-the-jabs/

The most highly cited physician on the early treatment of COVID-19 has come out with an explosive new interview that blows the lid off the medical establishment's complicity in the unnecessary deaths of thousands.

Dr. Peter McCullough said these deaths have been facilitated by a false narrative bent on pushing an all-new, unproven "vaccine" for a disease that was highly treatable.

He said the alleged "Covid-19" "virus" is a bioweapon, and the vaccines represent "phase two" of that bioweapon.

"As this, in a sense, bioterrorism phase one was rolled out, it was really all about keeping the population in fear and in isolation and preparing them to accept the vaccine, which appears to be phase two of a bioterrorism operation," McCullough said in a June 11, 2021, webinar with German attorney Reiner Fuellmich and several other doctors.

'Both the respiratory "virus" and the "vaccine" delivered to the human body the spike protein, the gain of function target of this bioterrorism research.'

'Now I can't come out and say all this on national TV today or at any time,' he continued. 'But what we had learned over time is that we could no longer communicate with government agencies. We actually couldn't even communicate with our propagandised colleagues in major medical centres, all of which appear to be under a spell, almost as if they are hypnotized right now.'

He did not hold back in his criticism of his colleagues in the medical community.

'And doctors, good doctors, are doing unthinkable things, like injecting biologically active messenger RNA that produces this pathological spike protein into pregnant women. I think when the doctors wake up from their trance, they're going to be shocked to think what they've done to people.'

McCullough was professor of medicine and vice chief of internal medicine at Baylor University and also taught at Texas A&M University. He is an epidemiologist, cardiologist and internist and has testified before the Texas State Senate related to "COVID-19" treatments. He holds the distinction of being the most widely cited physician in the treatment of "COVID-19" with more than 600 citations in the National Library of Medicine.

'The first wave of the bioterrorism is a respiratory virus that spread across the world and affected relatively few people—about one percent of many populations—but generated great fear.'

He said the **virus targeted primarily people over 50 with multiple medical conditions. It poses almost no risk to children.**

He said 85 percent of the more than 600,000 U.S. deaths could have been prevented with a multi-drug treatment given in the early to mid-point of the disease.

Instead, people were told to stay home and not return to the hospital unless their symptoms got worse, such as severe breathing problems. By then it was too late for many. **They were placed on ventilators and died.**

The vast majority of doctors jumped in lockstep to follow these erroneous "guidelines" handed down by the World Health Organisation and the U.S. Centre for Disease Control. Those guidelines neglected to place any focus on the treatment of sick patients and, from the beginning, as early as April 2020, started emphasizing the need for a vaccine as the only real hope of beating back the virus.

The federal Vaccine Adverse Event Reporting System [VAERS] logged 5,993 reports of deaths of people injected with the "COVID" "vaccine" between Dec. 14, 2020, and June 11, 2021 – **only 6 months**. **That's more than all the deaths reported to VAERS from all other vaccines combined over the last 22 years.**

We repeat to ensure the gravity of that statement is not lost:

The USA federal Vaccine Adverse Event Reporting System [VAERS] logged 5,993 reports of deaths of people injected with the "COVID" "vaccine" between Dec. 14, 2020, and June 11, 2021 - **only 6 months**. **That's more than all the deaths reported to VAERS from all other vaccines combined over the last 22 years.**

For those readers with an interest in Probability Theory, a reasonable estimate would result in the probability of the above happening is perhaps one in three existences of the Universe i.e. 1 in 14*3 Bn years namely 1 in 42Bn years. So, for those of us who believe in re-incarnation, then if you can plan your next life to occur in 42Bn years' time you may, or you may not, witness this preposterous circumstance that those of us actually alive and thinking today, have unfortunately already experienced.

But these numbers, as shocking as they are, don't scratch the surface of the actual number of dead Americans, said McCullough.

'We have now a whistle-blower inside the CMS, and we have two whistle-blowers in the CDC. ***We think we have 50,000 dead Americans.*** *Fifty thousand deaths.* ***So, we actually have more deaths due to the vaccine per day than certainly any viral illness by far. It's basically propagandized bioterrorism by injection.****'*

These numbers have most probably been replicated, per capita, proportionately all over the world since most countries used the same policies that were driven worldwide by pan-global organisations such as WHO, UN, WEF. Certainly, they have most probably been replicated in most countries in Europe and in UK.

McCullough added that ***'every single thing that was done in public health in response to the pandemic made it worse.'***

He said the suppression of early COVID treatments, such as hydroxychloroquine and especially Ivermectin, ***'was tightly linked to the development of a "vaccine".'***

Without the suppression of the already-available treatments, the government would not have been able to "legally" grant Emergency Use Authorisation to the three vaccines rushed to market in the USA by Moderna, Pfizer and Johnson and Johnson. However, since these treatments were readily available and known to genuine practitioners of medicine, the Emergency Use Authorisation for the three vaccines rushed to market was most probably an unlawful instrument.

Note that **'the suppression of the already-available treatments'** is a thorough, very serious and irrevocable breach of the Hippocratic Oath which is used to ensure the required high quality of ethics in Medicine and related subjects. This breach, if fully investigated, would lead to the suspension of practice licenses for every Doctor in the world where the Hippocratic Oath is in force. A rough estimate would be that in excess of 90% of Doctors world-wide would have their licenses revoked because of their un-ethical practices under the "Covid19" "pandemic".

In the case of Moderna, the U.S. government is co-patent holder through the National Institutes of Health, a clear conflict of interest, and confidential documents reveal Moderna sent a coronavirus mRNA vaccine candidate was sent to a US University in December 2019, **weeks before "Covid-19" was allegedly known to even exist**.

Ref: The above underlined statement is the Hyperlink to The Report – June 18th 2021

'I published basically the only two papers that teach doctors how to treat "COVID-19" at home to prevent hospitalisation and death…If treated early, it results in an 85 percent reduction in hospitalisations and death,' McCullough said.

So not only were the vaccines rolled out unnecessarily by suppressing already available, effective treatments, but the FDA and CDC are now covering up tragic numbers of deaths caused by their experimental, non-clinically trialled most probably unlawful, mRNA injections.

It is clear from the evidence of Dr Peter McCullough above, Dr Wagh, Dr Bhakdi, Dr Reiner Fuellmich et al that "Covid19" was not the result of a natural virus but the globally coordinated actions of very few, very powerful people to orchestrate a totally fake global "pandemic". The reasons for this and the resulting damage caused are explained in Chapter 14.

'We broke through to the people, and the people who got sick with "COVID" called in to get medications from mail-order distribution pharmacies. So, without the government even knowing what went on, we crushed the epidemic here in the United States towards the end of December and January [2020/2021].'

'We basically took care of the pandemic with about 500 doctors and telemedicine services. And to this day we treat about 25 percent of the US COVID-19 population that actually are at high risk, over age 50 with medical problems or present with severe symptoms. And we basically handled the pandemic, and at the same time we've tried to keep ourselves above the political fray.'

McCullough said his focus has recently turned to the unnecessary and dangerous injections – refer to subsequent chapters.

'We are working to change the public view of the "vaccine". The public initially accepted the "vaccine" and we had to kind of slowly turn the ship. Now, in the U.S. the rates of "vaccination" have been dropping since April 8* [2021]. *Most of the "vaccination" centres are empty.'

McCullough further stated:

'We have a lot going on in the United States. ***We are engaging more and more attorneys.'***

CHAPTER 6

CONFIDENCE TRICK 6: "COVID19" "VACCINES" ARE VACCINES – THEY ARE NOT

UNDERSTAND THESE KEY POINTS ABOUT THE "COVID" SHOTS:

- The experimental COVID shots are not traditional vaccines. They fall in the FDA regulatory category of gene-therapy agents. The mRNA and DNA are carried into our cells and alter our body's DNA to trigger production of the synthetic spike proteins and disrupt our normal immune system responses.
- This new technology, never used in vaccines before, triggers the body to make uncontrolled amounts of the spike proteins that led to unique reactions in the body not seen with traditional vaccines. These three reactions are primarily caused by the synthetic spike protein and by the lipid nanoparticle coating used to carry the mRNA or DNA into the body's cells to alter our own DNA.

- An exaggerated inflammatory response, causing damage to critical organs. In its most serious form, this is called cytokine storm.
- An exaggerated blood-clotting response, leading to multiple blood clots (thrombi) in the lungs, brain, kidneys, intestines and other critical organs. These blood clots can occur in both veins and arteries, which is unusual and potentially life-threatening if not treated rapidly.
- Vaccine-induced Acquired Immune Deficiency Syndrome (VI-AIDS). This means you are more susceptible to all kinds of illness outbreaks - viral, bacterial and fungal, as well as new cancers and recurrence of existing cancers.

Ref: https://www.truthforhealth.org/wp-content/uploads/2022/05/2022-VaccineInjury TreatmentGuide_4-29-22-FINAL.pdf

©Truth For Health Foundation 2022, a 501(c)(3) public charity. Provided as an educational resource

Luc Montagnier, Nobel laureate in medicine for discovering HIV

Quote:

'These "vaccines" are poisons. They are not real vaccines. The mRNA allows its message to be transcribed throughout the body, uncontrollably. No one can say for each of us where these messages will go. This is therefore a terrible unknown.'

'The 3 vaccines Pfizer, AstraZeneca, Moderna contain a sequence identified by Information Technology as transformation into a prion. There is therefore a known risk to human health.'

Ref: Appendix I – p18 PDF Download File

Dr Michael McDowell

Quotes:

'These [Covid19] *vaccines have never been used on the human population before. They are tools of "Frankenstein Technology" a "mystery" concoction – a Bio-Weapon – the spike protein* [they contain] *is a pathogen and it will damage you.'*

'The "vaccines" create vaccine induced antibodies; the vaccinated are then helpless against the [Covid19] *variants. This is called 'viral immune escape'.'*

Ref: https://rumble.com/embed/vonrmq/

Ref: Dr Richard Fleming PhD, MD, JD Distinguished Physician & Doctor of Law USA, Author:

'Is Covid-19 a Bioweapon? A Scientific and Forensic Investigation' – The Interview

Ref: https://australiaoneparty.com/truth-about-covid-coming-out-now/ for all Dr Richard Fleming quotations

Ref: 'Is Covid-19 a Bioweapon? A Scientific and Forensic Investigation (Children's Health Defense)' a hardback book by Dr Richard Fleming PhD, MD, JD published 7th September 2021

Dr Richard Fleming quote:

The "Sars-Cov2/Covd19" "vaccine":

1. Does not prevent you from getting infected from "Sars-Cov2/Covd19"
2. Does not reduce the number of "Covid19" cases
3. Does not prevent you from transmitting "Covid19"
4. There is no significant reduction in the number who get sick, "vaccinated" or NOT "vaccinated"

Unquote:

If this so called "vaccine" does not do what true vaccines are supposed to do i.e.

1. Prevent you from getting infected from "Sars-Cov2/Covd19"
2. Reduce the number of "Covid19" cases
3. Prevent you from transmitting "Covid19"
4. Achieve a significant reduction in the number who get sick by being "vaccinated"

Then it is NOT a vaccine because it demonstrably does not achieve exactly that that vaccines are meant to achieve! The "vaccines" DO NOT WORK!

"Sars-Cov2/Covd19" "vaccines" are not true "vaccines" – they are Bioweapons which will be clearly demonstrated in this book. Record DEATHS REPORTED by Insurance Companies.

Dr Richard Fleming quote:

'mRNA/DNA "vaccines" – Pfizer, Moderna etc. injected into people for just one type of spike protein only and not the rest of the "virus" does not give the person injected the full protection of potential forthcoming variants' [that a true vaccine strives to achieve].

'Antibody repression takes place.' Unquote

People injected have no protection from the forthcoming variants and consequently got sick from those variants. There are now potentially hundreds of variants of "Sars-Cov2/Covd19" throughout the world.

Ref: https://www.ecdc.europa.eu/en/covid-19/variants-concern

Dr Richard Fleming quote:

'The lack of protection against variants is clearly shown in the data from Israel, one of the most vaccinated countries in the world where multiple vaccinated patients are still being infected by "Sars-Cov2/Covd19" variants. Similarly, it is also shown in USA data.'

'You don't keep repeating the thing that does not work. All the evidence shows there is no statistical benefit for using these "vaccines". The mass "vaccination" has caused significant adverse side effects. These "vaccines" have done nothing to solve the problem.'

'The "vaccinations" need to be stopped.'

'The companies need to be held accountable.'

'The reasons why all these Treaties and Codes that we should abide by, but are being abused, needs to be addressed.'

'The gain of function research needs to be stopped.'

'We need to hold the people accountable who are responsible for doing this. They have violated the 'Biological Weapons Treaty'. They have violated 'The Nuremberg Code.'"

World-renowned vaccine developer Geert Vanden Bossche MVD, PhD warns that these **injections destroy the body's immune system**, making the vaccinated vulnerable for every new variant of the disease.

Ref: https://stopworldcontrol.com/downloads/en/vaccines/vaccinereport.pdf

He also says:

'Mass vaccination campaigns during a pandemic of highly infectious variants fail to control viral transmission. Instead of contributing to building herd immunity, they dramatically delay natural establishment of herd immunity. This is why the ongoing universal vaccination campaigns are absolutely detrimental to public and global health.'

The Nobel prize winner in medicine Dr. Luc Montagnier sounds the alarm that these vaccines are creating dangerous new variants. And in Israel the statistics show clearly a dramatic increase in "Covid" deaths once immunizations started (see earlier in this report). The **Israeli Prime Minister Naftali Bennet even says that the people who are most at risk now, are those who received two doses of the vaccine**.

In the island nation Seychelles there were hardly any "Covid" deaths, but once they started vaccinating the population, the deaths increased a hundred-fold.

True vaccines do not do what is reported above. **However, Bioweapons do!**

Anthony Fauci also made it crystal clear: ***'the CDC is considering mask mandates for the vaccinated', 'the vaccinated increasingly test positive for "Covid", therefor they will need to keep wearing masks', 'the vaccinated still need to avoid eating in restaurants', and 'the vaccinated carry the Delta variant as much as the unvaccinated'.***

So according to Fauci the vaccines do more or less nothing to stop the "virus"!

Yet he insists on mandating these useless injections for travel!

True vaccines do not do nothing useful!

The same was publicly stated by **the UK's Prime Minister Boris Johnson**, who said:

'Can I now meet my friends and family members indoors if they are vaccinated? There I am afraid the answer is no, because we're not yet at that stage, we're still very much in the world where you can meet friends and family outdoors, under the rule of six, or two households. And even if your friends and family members may be vaccinated, the vaccines are not giving 100% protection and that's why we need to be cautious.

Boris Johnson, as one would expect, is wildly and widely off the mark - the "vaccines" give no protection at all. Indeed, they are very harmful and can kill. Bioweapons tend to be harmful. That is their raison d'etre.

A research article published in 'Trends in Internal Medicine' by Dr. J. Bar Classen MD, is titled: 'US "COVID-19" "Vaccines" Proven to Cause More Harm than Good Based on Pivotal Clinical Trial Data Analysed Using the Proper Scientific Endpoint, states:

'All* ["COVID-19" "Vaccines"] *Cause Severe Morbidity'

Dr. Carrie Madej investigated vaccine vials from Moderna and Johnson & Johnson under a microscope with 400x magnification. What she saw shocked her ... **In both vials there was a living organism with tentacles. This creature moves around and lifts itself up.**

The sight of this and the thought that these unknown, octopus-like creatures are being injected into millions of children worldwide, caused Dr. Madej to weep.

Dr. Madej also observed pieces of graphene in the vials, as well as self-assembling nanoparticles. The particles moved towards one another and formed more complex structures. The same was revealed by Dr. Zandre Botha from South Africa. She studied several vaccine vials using a variety of methods, and what she found is simply too bizarre for words. Just like Dr. Carrie Madej she saw complex self-assembling nanobots.

Ref: https://stopworldcontrol.com/downloads/en/vaccines/vaccinereport.pdf

Dr. Madej horrendous images pp 17,18 of the above report.

What kind of diabolical agenda is secretly being rolled out, by injecting these kinds of self-assembling nanobots into the bodies of millions of people? And why are so many news agencies, and so-called fact-checkers doing overtime to deny these apparent, undeniable findings? What is really the purpose of these injections, that are so forcefully being imposed onto all of humanity? And why are all the governments worldwide collaborating with this plan? There clearly is a nefarious agenda behind covertly injecting this kind of nanotechnology into humanity. What is it? Who dares to ask these questions, and find the answers?

The world-renowned biophysicist Andreas Kalcker has discovered that the "vaccines" contain large amounts of **graphene oxide** (up to 95%). He warns that the graphene oxide injected into humans is **altering their electromagnetic field**, which **disrupts the normal functioning of their organs.**

'What we are concerned about is the side effects it has. This isn't described in medicine, but it's described in my field, biophysics. What happens? The body needs its electro molecular capabilities to work. The heart beats because there's a magnetic field that creates, subsequently, the electricity for pumping and everything else. **Graphene is completely altering our electromagnetic field, something that has never happened before.** What we're seeing is something 'in vivo' with some dramatic effects. We have been watching a lot of videos of people who are dying after being vaccinated. You see people spasming. These spasms have, for example, very specific frequencies, and they are the same in all kinds of spasms.'

'These spasms indicate that there is a disruption of the human electromagnetic fields.'

The presence of graphene oxide, among other toxic materials like aluminum, LNP capsids, PEG and parasites in the vaccines was further confirmed by Dr. Robert Young. The Scientist's Club also released a report with microphotographic evidence of nanoparticles in the "vaccines". Major revelations on what is in the "CoV-2-19" vaccines, with the use of electron, pHase, dark field, bright field and other types of microscopy from the original research of Dr. Robert Young and his scientific team, confirming what the La Quinta Columna researchers found - **toxic nanometallic content with magneticotoxic, cytotoxic and genotoxic effects, as well as identified life-threatening parasites.**

18 Scientist Worldwide Test ALL Available "Vaccines"
Studies led by Dr Poornima Wagh.

- Our group of 18 scientists, currently as of August 23, 2022, started out as a group of only 4 scientists in late January 2021 on the testing of the "Covid19" injections. Collectively as more scientists joined the group through 2021, **18 scientists have now tested 2305 vials** (as of August 23, 2022) of the following "Covid19" injections from all over the world since November/December 2020 when the injections first rolled out:
- 1. Pfizer/BioNtech/Cominarty, 2. Moderna, 3. Johnson & Johnson (J&J), 4. Novavax, 5. AstraZeneca, 6. Sinopharm (China), 7. Sinovac (China), 8. Covishield (Homegrown version of AstraZeneca made in India), 9. Soberana 02 (Cuba), 10. Pasto Covac (Iran), 11. CanSino (China), 12. ZifiVax (China)

Study Locations & Product Numbers Tested

- **United States**: 86 Pfizer jabs, 41 Moderna jabs, 25 Johnson & Johnson jabs, 3 Novavax jabs.
- **Argentina**: 138 Pfizer jabs, 122 Moderna jabs, 50 Sinopharm jabs, 46 AstraZeneca jabs.
- **Australia**: 141 AstraZeneca jabs, 112 Pfizer jabs, 90 Moderna jabs, 1 Novavax jab.
- **New Zealand**: 120 Pfizer jabs (including the pediatric shots), 78 Astra Zeneca jabs, 25 Johnson & Johnson jabs, 1 Novavax jab.

Dr Wagh's Summary of the Contents and Adverse
Effects of the "Vaccines"
They are
CHEMICAL WEAPONS!!

- **These INJECTIONS are deadly CHEMICAL COCKTAILS, <u>NOT a bioweapon, but a chemical weapon</u>. The INGREDIENTS are as follows:**
- 1. Adjuvants (which are preservatives which is mostly Aluminum hydroxide, and a few others), 2. Sucrose (sugar), 4. Sodium Chloride (salt), 5. Water, 6. Synthetic lipid nano particles such as PEG and SM 102, 7. Hydrogel (Polymer Nanoparticle called PNP), 8.Trillions of nano particles of reduced graphene oxide, 9. Trillions of particles of nano particulate of heavy metal contamination.

ADVERSE EFFECTS:

- Synthetic lipid nano particles such as PEG (Polyethylene Glycol) and SM 102 are highly inflammatory substances for the body, sometimes causing the body to go into anaphylactic shock. They are highly carcinogenic and cancer-causing substances.
- There was MASSIVE contamination in the Covid 19 injections through heavy metal particulate such as tungsten, chromium, iron, sodium (highly electro conductive), strontium, magnesium, gold and silver nano particulates, lead, antimony, aluminum, tin and many others. This heavy metal sludge is very stable and is attracted to fat tissue in the body and gets deposited there causing repeated irritation and inflammation in the body leading to disease and degeneration of the body.
- Reduced graphene oxide because of its positive magnetic and electric charge literally SHORT CIRCUITS the insides of the human body causing massive inflammation and degeneration of tissues. Graphene is known to get attracted to the negatively charged organs, blood vessels and nervous system and completely damage the electrical activity of the body. Hence, we're seeing a whopping increase in myocarditis, pericarditis, strokes, clots, heart attacks, and seizures in vaccinated people. The electrical activity in the body is getting completely disrupted, and the body in most cases responds with massive systemic inflammation causing eventual degeneration and death.

CONCLUSIONS:

- Since ALL the injections tested all over the world were nearly identical with the same ingredients list of chemicals, heavy metals, hydrogel, synthetic lipid nanos and trillions of particles of REDUCED graphene oxide under different brand names such as Pfizer, Moderna, Sinopharm etc. with NO BIOLOGICS in the injections, it is safe to say this injection and booster scheme was deployed as a depopulation tactic and thereafter technocratic totalitarian control of the leftover population on the planet.
- This is why boosters are given, as each successive wave of injections weakens the body progressively and cuts life spans into a fraction after each dose. This is also why the parasites in charge masquerading as government are encouraging mixing and matching of boosters for all the injections, because every single injection for Covid is IDENTICAL and has the same ingredients made to kill and maim the body.

Ref: https://rumble.com/v1gd241-dr.-lee-merritt-and-poornima-wagh-phd.html

CHAPTER 7

CONFIDENCE TRICK 7: "COVID19" "VACCINES" WERE SAFE – THEY ARE NOT

'The USA Vaccine Adverse Event Reporting System 'VAERS' reports more deaths and adverse side effects were caused by the "Covid19" "Vaccines" than <u>ALL</u> other vaccines together, used for the last 30 years!'

Dr Richard Fleming PhD, MD, JD
Distinguished Physician & Doctor of Law USA

"COVID19" - UNPRECEDENTED!

Many aspects of "Covid-19" and subsequent "vaccine" development are unprecedented for a vaccine deployed for use in the general population. Some of these includes the following:

1. First to use PEG (polyethylene glycol) in an injection
2. First Coronavirus vaccine ever attempted in humans
3. First to use mRNA vaccine technology against an infectious agent
4. First time Moderna has brought any product to market
5. First to have public health officials telling those receiving the vaccination to expect an adverse reaction
6. First to be implemented publicly with nothing more than preliminary efficacy data, no long-term safety data
7. First vaccine to make no clear claims about reducing infections, transmissibility, or deaths
8. First injection of genetically modified polynucleotides in the general population

Here is the <u>PFIZER</u> data <u>FORCIBLY</u> released under <u>COURT ORDER</u>:

Was there any BENEFIT of the COVID shots in the drug companies' clinical trial studies?

- No evidence of reduced spread to others.
- No evidence of reduced hospitalizations or reduced deaths.
- Evidence that taking the COVID shot increased the risk of death to trial participants by 50%.

- Evidence that taking the COVID shot impairs your immune response, called the Vaccine-induced Acquired Immune Deficiency Syndrome. This makes you more susceptible to a variety of other viral, bacterial, and fungal infections, as well as increased risk of cancer (new or recurrence of existing).

UNDERSTAND THESE KEY POINTS ABOUT THE COVID SHOTS:

- ➢ **The experimental COVID shots are not traditional vaccines.** They fall in the FDA regulatory category of **gene-therapy agents**. The mRNA and DNA are carried into our cells and **alter our body's DNA** to trigger production of the synthetic spike proteins and disrupt our normal immune system responses.
- ➢ **This new technology, never used in vaccines before,** triggers the **body to make uncontrolled amounts of the spike proteins** that led to unique reactions in the body not seen with traditional vaccines. These three reactions are primarily caused by the synthetic spike protein and by the lipid nanoparticle coating used to carry the mRNA or DNA into the body's cells **to alter our own DNA**.
- **An exaggerated inflammatory response, causing damage to critical organs.** In its most serious form, this is called **cytokine storm**.
- **An exaggerated blood-clotting response,** leading to **multiple blood clots (thrombi) in the lungs, brain, kidneys, intestines and other critical organs**. These blood clots can occur in both veins and arteries, which is unusual and potentially life-threatening if not treated rapidly.
- **Vaccine-induced Acquired Immune Deficiency Syndrome (VI-AIDS).** This means you are **more susceptible to all kinds of illness outbreaks - viral, bacterial, and fungal, as well as new cancers and recurrence of existing cancers**.

What groups of people are at the greatest RISKS of adverse effects with taking the "COVID" shot?

- People who had "COVID2 or suspected "COVID" (with positive antibodies for COVID) are already immune and risks of serious adverse reactions are much higher.
- People with past allergic or other adverse reactions to vaccines.
- People with allergies to PEG (polyethylene glycol).
  mRNA vaccines use PEG to stabilize lipid nanoparticles. About 70% of people have antibodies to PEG, which can cause a life-threatening reaction (anaphylaxis)
- ALL CHILDREN
- ALL women and men of childbearing age

- People with chronic cardiac, respiratory, and endocrine conditions
- People with a history of autoimmune disorders
- People at risk for, or who have a history of cancer

What are the reported SIDE EFFECTS, and COMPLICATIONS? (Ref: Go to https://openvaers.com/covid-data)

There are now over 1,800,000 adverse events reported in VAERS related to uptake of the "COVID" shot, including over 25,000 deaths and over 140,000 hospitalizations

- General symptoms such as fever, headaches, fatigue, weakness, muscle pain, swollen lymph nodes
- Nervous system effects: changes in sensation, Bell's Palsy, imbalance with walking, severe headaches, brain lesions, micro blood clots in the brain, changes in thinking and memory and seizures, Lewey body dementia, rapidly progressive dementia (Jacob Creutzfeldt), flareup of multiple sclerosis and other neurodegenerative diseases such as ALS, Parkinson's
- Eyes: blood clots, vision loss/blindness, blurred vision, acuity loss, glaucoma, macular degeneration
- Ears: ringing in the ears (tinnitus), loss of hearing, dizziness/vertigo, loss of balance
- Cardiovascular system effects such as racing heart, chest pain, heart attacks, heart failure, myocarditis and pericarditis (especially in young people and athletes), low and abnormal red and white blood cells, low platelets, bleeding disorders, abnormal clotting
- Respiratory system effects such as changes in the lung tissue, asthmatic changes, shortness of breath, difficulty breathing with activity and recurring infections (pneumonia)
- Gastric system effects such a gastric bleeding, irritable bowel syndrome, gastric ulcers
- Immune deficiency syndrome leading to recurrent infections with atypical organisms or dormant viruses like Shingles, impaired cancer surveillance functions leading to increase in new and aggressive cancers, recurrence of cancers previously in remission.
- Autoimmune disorders worsening: Crohn's disease, pernicious anemia, autoimmune thyroiditis, rheumatoid arthritis, Lupus, and others
- Skin changes: petechiae, increase in bruising, unusual rashes, shingles outbreaks, painful hives, skin cancers, wounds that do not heal
- Reproductive system effects such as
  - Women: miscarriages; deaths of mothers, deaths of nursing babies after mother vaccinated, abnormal bleeding, menstrual problems
  - Men: testicular pain/inflammation

Ref – for the four text boxes above: https://www.truthforhealth.org/wp-content/uploads/2022/05/2022-VaccineInjuryTreatmentGuide_4-29-22-FINAL.pdf

This is a very good report. The reader is encouraged to read it in full.

Furthermore as shown in the previous chapter, Dr Wagh has exposed how damaging these "vaccines" are with the results of her extensive study project:

ALL "COVID" "VACCINE" ADVERSE EFFECTS:

- Synthetic lipid nano particles such as PEG (Polyethylene Glycol) and SM 102 are highly inflammatory substances for the body, sometimes causing the body to go into anaphylactic shock. They are highly carcinogenic and cancer-causing substances.
- There was MASSIVE contamination in the Covid 19 injections through heavy metal particulate such as tungsten, chromium, iron, sodium (highly electro conductive), strontium, magnesium, gold and silver nano particulates, lead, antimony, aluminum, tin and many others. This heavy metal sludge is very stable and is attracted to fat tissue in the body and gets deposited there causing repeated irritation and inflammation in the body leading to disease and degeneration of the body.
- Reduced graphene oxide because of its positive magnetic and electric charge literally SHORT CIRCUITS the insides of the human body causing massive inflammation and degeneration of tissues. Graphene is known to get attracted to the negatively charged organs, blood vessels and nervous system and completely damage the electrical activity of the body. Hence, we're seeing a whopping increase in myocarditis, pericarditis, strokes, clots, heart attacks, and seizures in vaccinated people. The electrical activity in the body is getting completely disrupted, and the body in most cases responds with massive systemic inflammation causing eventual degeneration and death.

SHOCK ANNOUNCEMENT BY UK NHS (National Health Service)
UK NHS HAS NO RECORD OF PROOF OF EXISTANCE OF SARs-COV-2
and
NO PROOF THAT "COVID?" "VACCINES ARE SAFE! 25th Nov. 2022

See Appendix II

Ref: https://www.covid19compensation2022.com/HOT-NEWS

SHOCK ANNOUNCEMENT BY UK GMC (General Medical Council)
UK NHS HAS NO RECORD OF PROOF OF EXISTANCE OF SARs-COV-2
and
NO PROOF THAT "COVID?" "VACCINES ARE SAFE! 6th Dec. 2022

See Appendix II

Ref: https://www.covid19compensation2022.com/HOT-NEWS

Dr Michael McDowell

Quotes:

'These* [Covid19] *"vaccines" have never been used on the human population before. They are tools of "Frankenstein Technology" a "mystery" concoction – a Bio-Weapon – the spike protein* [they contain] *is a pathogen and it will damage you.'

'The "vaccines" create "vaccine" induced antibodies; the vaccinated are then helpless against the* [Covid19] *variants. This is called 'viral immune escape'.'

Ref: https://rumble.com/embed/vonrmq/

Ref: Dr Richard Fleming PhD, MD, JD Author:

***'Is Covid-19 a Bioweapon? A Scientific and Forensic Investigation'* – The Interview**

Ref: https://australiaoneparty.com/truth-about-covid-coming-out-now/ for all Dr Richard Fleming quotations.

In this very important and very serious interview referenced above, **Dr Richard Fleming swears under oath that "Sars-Cov2" is a Bioweapon** (he is a Doctor of Law) and by de facto implication it is **not a natural virus**, which has been conclusively demonstrated in previous chapters of this book. From this statement we can reasonably and fairly deduce that "Sars-Cov2" was constructed by human beings for the purpose of doing harm to other human beings. This is supported by the fact that ***'The USA Vaccine Adverse Event Reporting System 'VAERS' reports more deaths and adverse side effects were caused by the "Covid19" "Vaccines" than ALL other vaccines together, used for the last 30 years!'***

However, Health Authorities worldwide (**including the NHS UK**) and Big Pharma – the suppliers of these "vaccines" – Pfizer, AstraZeneca, Moderna and Johnson & Johnson claimed that the "vaccines" were safe. They also made this very rash, utter nonsense claim even though the "vaccines" had not undergone full clinical trials, a process that usually takes 7 to 10 years.

VAERS was established in 1990 in USA, the Vaccine Adverse Event Reporting System (VAERS) is a national early warning system to detect possible safety problems in U.S.-licensed vaccines. VAERS is co-managed by the Centers for Disease Control and Prevention (CDC) and the U.S. Food and Drug Administration (FDA). VAERS accepts and analyses reports of adverse events (possible side effects) after a person has received a vaccination.

Unbelievably, in the VAERS system in the USA, there is no specific code for "Sars-Cov2"/"Covid19", whereas there is for other vaccines. One is simply bounced from one computer message to another. How can this possibly be the case for what is claimed to be an enormously threatening "pandemic"? Is the access to this important VAERS system for the data relating to "Sars-Cov2"/"Covid19" deliberately made difficult for researchers? Do the health authorities in USA the CDC and FDA not truly want the people to know the TRUTH about the adverse reactions? Do the Government and Health Authorities in USA and world-wide not want the people of USA and the world to know the truth that **"Sars-Cov2" is a Bioweapon** constructed by laboratories in USA and Wuhan, China? It is clearly very obvious that they would not want the truth to be known. Hence the global blanket, in lockstep propaganda narrative with not one single mainstream news outlet offering a scintilla of information that was in any microscopic way not finely tuned to the global one-dimensional false narrative.

In the interview Dr. Fleming goes on to state that in 2010 scientists in Wuhan, China KNEW that viruses in bats could NOT affect humans. Research proved this. Yet the global blanket, in military-type lockstep, propaganda narrative with not one single main stream news outlet offering a scintilla of information that was in any microscopic way not finely tuned to the global one dimensional false narrative that pushed the view that the "Sars-Cov2" "virus" emanated from bats in a market in Wuhan, China.

There were at least two gain of function elements to the "Sars-Cov2" "virus". One was the PRA insert the second was the HIV protein insert.

Refer to Dr Poornima Wagh Chapter 1:

Dr Poornima Wagh, Researcher, 2 PhDs in Virology and Immunology, Santa Barbara, CA, USA

Quote:

***"How do you find HIV spike proteins in a 'NOVEL' virus genome? You don't, it's called FRAUD"* [What has been called, by WHO etc. "Sars-Cov-2" IS NOT a virus!]**

The HIV insert causes prions. Prions are very dangerous; people die from prion diseases. Refer to Luc Montagnier below as previously quoted:

Luc Montagnier, Nobel laureate in medicine for discovering HIV: quote:

'These "vaccines" are poisons. They are not real vaccines. As a doctor I knew 21 people who received 2 doses of Pfizer vaccine, there is another person who received Moderna. The 21 died of Creutzfeldt-Jakob disease caused by prions. The 3 vaccines Pfizer, AstraZeneca, Moderna contain a sequence identified by Information Technology as transformation into a prion. There is therefore a known risk to human health.'

Dr Fleming, quote ***'This is playing GOD!'***

Dr Fleming, quote ***'There would have been NO "pandemic" if this "virus" had not been deliberately released"***

To be certain that this very important point has not been missed, to repeat:

Dr Fleming, quote ***'There would have been NO "pandemic" if this "virus" had not been deliberately released"***

Putting together all the information contained in this book it is clear that the release of this constructed man-made "virus" was a deliberate act.

Dr Fleming, quote:

'Dr Fauci,* Medical Advisor to President of USA lied when he stated that the USA Authorities were not involved in *gain of function research*. USA medical authorities National Institutes of Health 'NIH' and National Institute of Allergy Infectious Diseases 'NIAID' *have admitted it*. If such violations of the truth are undertaken by a person who has been sworn into official office in USA, then it constitutes violation of oath and therefore the person may be *put on trial for treason*.' [It is plausible, when one takes into consideration all the evidence available, in particular Dr Fauci's emails released to a Senate Hearing in USA, that Dr Fauci may be susceptible to trial for treason.]

Dr Fleming, quote

'Gain of function spike protein is a Bioweapon. Why would you replicate that function and put it in a "vaccine"?

The "vaccines" go ALL over the body! **[They break the blood-brain barrier and enter the brain]** ***They cause blood clots! The injected body is infected with billions of particles of*** **[harmful]** ***virus material'***

'Pfizer and the other pharmaceutical companies making these "vaccines" did not undertake animal studies on the effects of the "vaccines" before or after "emergency authorisation" was given. ***Independent studies on animals showed: damage to the brains and other body organs, prion diseases, inflammation or blood clotting, thrombotic diseases, real concerns about baby miscarriages, other health problems and deaths. The studies on animals have been very consistent on this.*** *This animal research should have been done* ***BEFORE*** *emergency use authorisation.* ***This violates any treaty and code that we have ever had as human beings. There was one time when trial studies were done on human beings BEFORE any trials on animals and those people guilty were prosecuted at The Nuremberg Trials*** **[Crimes Against Humanity, Nuremberg, Germany] in 1947!'**

The Nuremberg trials [supposedly] established that all of humanity would be guarded by an international legal shield and that even a Head of State would be held criminally responsible and punished for aggression and Crimes Against Humanity.

On the basis of the purpose of the Nuremberg trials outlined above, then presumably prosecutions will shortly commence against those responsible to ensure that the 'international legal shield' will be effective in protecting us from such evil!

Dr Fleming, quote:

'What happens if the "vaccines" get into the blood stream? We have looked at Pfizer, Moderna, Johnson & Johnson and have looked at the effect those "vaccines" have on the blood – the effects are almost immediate. Three slides from seven different patients with all three "vaccines" being tested show what happened. The blood samples were inspected under a microscope. In the first

image you can see the Pfizer"vaccine" that was added to the blood. The nice red blood cells carrying oxygen to the body. The grey cells next to the red ones are red cells originally but they are no longer red because they have been infected with the Pfizer "vaccine". This infection causes the blood cells to no longer be able to carry oxygen to the body. In the second slide you see the exact same thing in another patient; this is the Moderna "vaccine". The Johnson & Johnson "vaccines show the same thing in the third slide. When the blood cells are no longer red then the haemoglobin is no longer able to carry oxygen to the body. The haemoglobin molecule has been damaged or the membrane of the red blood cell has been damaged. ***This damage does not reverse.*** *'*

Ref: *https://australiaoneparty.com/truth-about-covid-coming-out-now/* - video interview

Slide 1, slide 2, slide 3 mentioned by Dr Fleming are shown and discussed at 40:20 – 41:30 mins:secs at the Ref: URL video interview immediately above.

'The other thing that we saw was that the blood begins to clump together. The red blood cells carry oxygen to the lungs and carbon dioxide from the lungs. This damage to the haemoglobin means that the ***blood cells cannot, most probably, even carry away the carbon dioxide – the waste product! No amount of these "vaccines" should have damaging effects on the patients' red blood cells.*** *This is a very simple study to carry out –* ***prove me wrong if you can!*** *However, you will not because these effects were found in repeatable, and repeated studies with a number of patients and various laboratories located in different places on the planet.'*

'We have known for a very long time ***where RNA or DNA is outside of a prion then this is very dangerous****. Red blood cells cannot do anything with genetic code that is entered into them. The lipid nanoparticles would simply merge with the red blood cells – the protein structure changes and the haemoglobin can no longer pick up the oxygen or the carbon dioxide.* ***This change is permanent. Important mechanisms in the anti-body creation in the "vaccinated" patient are suppressed.*** *'*

[lipids are any of a class of organic compounds that are fatty acids or their derivatives and are insoluble in water but soluble in organic solvents. They include many natural oils, waxes, and steroids. Lipid nanoparticles, are nanoparticles composed of lipids. They are a novel pharmaceutical drug delivery system, and a novel pharmaceutical formulation. A nanoparticle or ultrafine particle is usually defined as a particle of matter that is between 1 and 100 nanometres in diameter.]

[For example, the "Sars-Cov2/Covid19" "virus" is c. 100-160 Nano-meters in diameter – 100-160 meter*10^-9. This is very, very, very small – a metaphorical example would be that 1 nanometre would be the diameter of a marble resting on the North Pole in comparison to the size of the Earth. Now ask yourself why there are over 140 independent studies world-wide on the **non-effectiveness of masks** in their ability to prevent such a small particle, the "Sars-Cov2/Covid19" "virus" to pass through the mask. **In a brief sentence, masks are completely worthless in preventing "Covid19". If you have purchased any, then investigate suing under the Trade Descriptions Act 2011 (in UK).** See Chapter 9.]

Dr Fleming, quote:

'*When you have people at a FDA* [Food and Drug Administration USA] *meeting saying we need to vaccinate the children but we will not know what happens to them until we vaccinate them! That's the experimental phase of a Research Project.* ***It appears that our Governments do not have a problem experimenting on our elderly, on our Police Officers, on our First Response Staff, on our Doctors and Nurses, on our General Public and now apparently don't have a problem experimenting on our children'*** [Publicly voiced in interview August 2022]

[This experimentation has been happening all over the world since 2020. Surely this offence must at the very least be criminal negligence!]

Further Ref: **'Is Covid-19 a Bioweapon? A Scientific and Forensic Investigation (Children's Health Defense)'** a hardback book by Dr Richard Fleming PhD, MD, JD published 7th September 2021.

There is further evidence that the "Vaccines" are not safe in the many reports of them causing severe blood clots. Independent research has shown that many patients who took the "vaccines" have incurred very long, fibrous blood clots never previously seen by professional embalmers.

Ref: https://www.christianitydaily.com/articles/14923/20220214/veteran-embalmer-observes-increased-blood-clots-among-vaccinated-dead-people.htm

In addition, independent research has shown that there has been an enormous drop in birth-rate after the "vaccination" 'roll out' [the inoculations are not true vaccines, they are mRNA treatments per mRNA architecture - Dr Robert Malone, USA] from studies for Germany, UK, USA, Taiwan and others. The report shows that the drop in birth-rate is up to 26 Sigmas. **Meaning very highly improbable to have been caused by natural causes**. Causality suggests a link between "Covid19" "vaccinations" and the drop in birth-rate, which is the reported intention by the Evil300 as described in our Report.

Ref: https://truth613.substack.com/p/hashem-yeracheim-may-g-d-have-mercy

More evidence of Health Authorities malpractice comes from Thomas Renz USA:

Wave Of Evidence Damns Big Pharma: Accountability Coming for Medical Cabal

Thomas Renz, Attorney at Law, USA:

Quote:

"The FDA* [Federal and Drug Administration USA] *in October 2020 knew about the truth of Covd-19 "vaccines" being a global gene therapy experiment trial and lied about it."

The "Vaccine" Death Report

by

Dr David John Sorenson & Dr Vladimir Zelenko

Evidence of millions of deaths and serious adverse events resulting from the experimental "COVID-19" injections is given in the above report. Information such as: According to a CDC health fraud detection expert the **number of "vaccine" deaths in the U.S. is not 15,386 but somewhere between 80,000 and 160,000.**

Ref: https://stopworldcontrol.com/downloads/en/vaccines/vaccinereport.pdf

Furthermore, VAERS data from the American CDC shows that as of September 17, 2021, **already 726,963 people suffered adverse events**, including **stroke, heart failure, blood clots, brain disorders, convulsions, seizures, inflammations of brain & spinal cord, life-threatening allergic reactions, autoimmune diseases, arthritis, miscarriage, infertility, rapid-onset muscle weakness, deafness, blindness, narcolepsy, and cataplexy**.

It is Far Worse Than We Think

1. VAERS published 726,963 adverse events, including 15,386 deaths as of September 17, 2021
2. CDC fraud expert says that number of deaths is at least five times, and possibly ten times higher
3. A whistle-blower from the Centers for Medicare & Medicaid Service (CMS) revealed how almost 50,000 people died from the injections. They represent only 20% of the U.S. population, meaning that if this data is applied to the entire population 250,000 have died
4. 150,000 reports have been rejected or scrubbed by the VAERS system
5. The actual number of anaphylaxes is 50 to 120 times higher than claimed by the CDC
6. Everyone who dies before two weeks after the second injection, is not considered a vaccine death, which causes the majority of early vaccine deaths to be ignored
7. Moderna received over 300,000 reports of adverse events in only three months-time
8. The Lazarus Report shows that only 1% of adverse events is being reported by the public
9. The majority of the population is not aware of the existence of systems where they can report vaccine adverse events
10. Aggressive censorship and propaganda told the public that adverse events are rare, causing people to not understand how their health problems stem from past injections
11. The shaming and blaming of medical professionals who say anything against the vaccines, cause many in the medical community to avoid reporting adverse events
12. The fear of being held accountable after administering an injection that killed or disabled patients, further prevents medical personnel from reporting it

13. Having accepted financial incentives to promote, and administer the covid vaccines, also stops medical personnel from reporting adverse events
14. Profit driven vaccine manufacturers have every reason not to report the destruction their untested experimental products are causing
15. 250,000+ Facebook users comment about vaccine deaths and serious injuries

This alarming data leads world experts, like the Nobel Prize Winner in Medicine, Dr. Luc Montagnier, to issue a grave warning that we are currently facing the greatest risk of worldwide genocide, in the history of humanity. Even the inventor of the mRNA technology, Dr. Robert Malone, warns against these injections that are using his technology. The situation is so severe that former Pfizer vice president and chief scientist Dr. Mike Yeadon came forward to warn humanity for these extremely dangerous injections. One of his best known videos is titled ‘A Final Warning’. Another world renown scientist, Geert Vanden Bossche, former Head of Vaccine Development Office in Germany, and Chief Scientific Officer at Univac, also risks his name and career, by bravely speaking out against administration of the “Covid” shots. **The vaccine developer warns that the injections can compromise the immunity of the vaccinated, making them vulnerable to every new variant**. World War II holocaust survivors wrote to the European Medicines Agency demanding the “Covid19” injections to be stopped, which they consider to be a new holocaust.

Full details of the estimated true numbers of deaths and the true number of adverse side effects are dealt with in Chapter 11.

“Covid19” “Vaccines” are not Safe – Graphene Oxide and 5G

Ref: https://stopworldcontrol.com/downloads/en/vaccines/vaccinereport.pdf

As we all know, the goal of criminals is to always increase their power and wealth. They are never satisfied but continually crave more. Ultimately, they want to play ‘god’ over the whole world, where everybody will be their servant. To keep increasing their power, there is one thing they need: the blind obedience of the masses. Only a totally ignorant and utterly obedient population will collaborate with their plans. That’s why they have been buying the entire world’s mainstream news media, education systems, health care, and government agencies, etc. so they can use all of that to spread their brainwashing propaganda to every mind in every corner of the world. Still, they don’t stop here, as they are fully aware that not everybody believes everything on television. Therefore, their plan to gain 100% control over the minds of all of humanity has further developed. Recently their agenda has been voiced loud and clear by the Chilean president Sebastián Piñera. In a public speech, he bluntly announced to the entire nation:

‘Let’s hear what the leaders of the world launch in this community. It is the possibility that machines can read our thoughts and can even insert thoughts, insert feelings. 5G is a tremendous leap. It’s a cosmic leap, a Copernican leap, because really what 5G technology is going to mean is an even greater shift in our lives than all the previous technologies have meant. <u>It offers the possibility that machines can read our thoughts and can even insert thoughts, insert feelings.</u> That’s not just going to change life, it’s going to transform

it. 5G in the actual nervous system of our society, just like that. It is to modernize our state, to be a change that reaches every home in our country.'

After stealing our voices through censorship, stealing our votes through election fraud, stealing our money through ever-increasing taxes, **they will now steal our very own thoughts and feelings through 5G**. That will be the summit of their tyranny, as they will be able to impose the desired thoughts and feelings onto the whole world, so nobody will even be able to divert from their narrative anymore. Is that why Klaus Schwab [Chairman, World Economic Forum – WEF] so confidently states in his promotional videos about the near future:

Quote: **Klaus Schwab Chairman, World Economic Forum – WEF**

'<u>2030: You'll own nothing. And you will be happy. Whatever you want you'll rent</u>'

THE 'GREAT RESET' DANGER

<u>'GREAT RESET' ACTIVITY TIMELINE</u>

COVID19/VAX(Digital Vax Passport-partially achieved) ➡ GLOBAL DIGITAL ID (starting now)

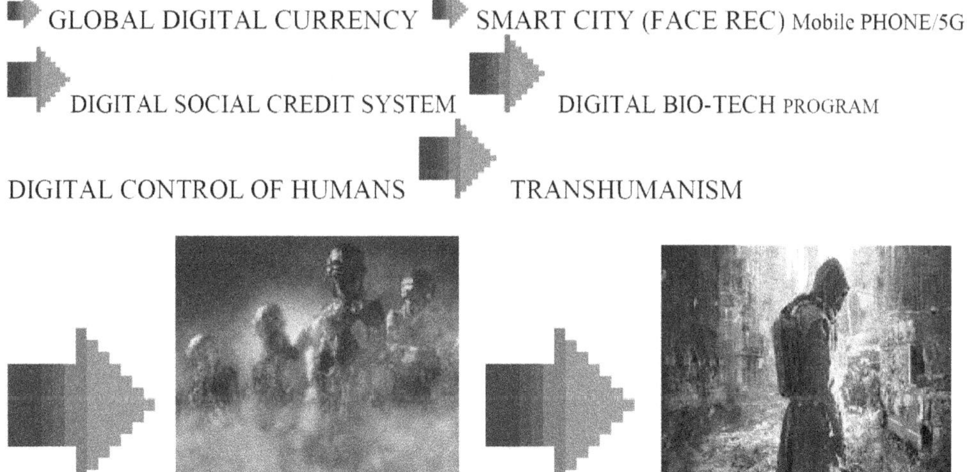

THE GLOBAL HUMANOID-ROBOT TOTALITARIAN DYSTOPIA

<u>Dr. Yuval Harari</u> advisor to Klaus Schwab WEF has endorsed this insanity on numerous occasions – see below:

Yuval Harari advisor to Klaus Schwab WEF World Economic Forum quote:

<u>'Governments and Corporations can hack Human Beings… Soul, Spirit, Free Will - in humans, that's over!!!'</u>

Ref: https://www.youtube.com/watch?v=NV0CtZga7qM

Dr Reiner Fuellmich – International Anti-Corporate Corruption Trial Lawyer – Chairman Corona Investigative Committee (Germany/World-Wide) Founder 'International Crime Investigative Committee' 'ICIC' and a world-renowned trial lawyer with almost three decades of experience in successfully suing large fraudulent corporations, such as Deutsche Bank, Volkswagen, etc. **stated that Dr Yuval Harari's statements were '<u>Pure Evil</u>!'**

Could it be that Klaus Schwab is referring to an artificially induced state of fake happiness created within the Humanoid-Robots that emanate from the fertile imagination of his henchman Dr Yuval Harari? What does this have to do with this vaccine report? It could be more than we are aware of right now. For 5G to be able to modify the thoughts and feelings of the population it requires another element: nanoparticles inside of the brains of people that receive and transmit the 5G signals.

<u>It turns out that the substance that is most efficient in communicating with 5G is the very substance that is massively present in the "Covid" injections: graphene oxide.</u>

And idiots all over the world claim that "Covid19" "vaccines" ARE SAFE!!

No substance on earth communicates better with 5G than graphene oxide, and no substance in existence is more **efficient in penetrating the human brain and manipulating human thoughts and feelings**, than **graphene**. One company that has been using graphene to manipulate the human brain, for medical purposes, is **IN BRAIN Neuro Electronics**. Their website states:

'We use graphene, the thinnest material known to man to build the new generation of neural interfaces for brain restoration to help patients around the world.'

The company highlights its technology as being able to 'read' a person's brain, detect specific neurological patterns, and then control that person's neurology to alter their brain function. It appears that the intention of INBRAIN is to merely help people with neurological disorders, but the reason they are mentioned here is to illustrate how graphene is indeed the ideal substance to alter the human brain. And again, it works better with 5G than anything else.

The fact that it [graphene] is present in the "Covid" "vaccines", is therefore highly disturbing, especially if we know what the agenda is of the world leaders, as described by the Chilean president:

'5G offers the possibility that machines can read our thoughts and can even insert thoughts, insert feelings.'

Do you really want your children and grandchildren to be raised in such a dystopian nightmare?

Another element we have to touch on, is the clear and public agenda of the globalists (Evil300) to end humanity as we know it and steer all of us into becoming cyborgs (over which they will have total control). This is clearly explained in the book of Klaus

Schwab 'The Fourth Industrial Revolution'. He strongly believes humans need to become one with machines, that are fully connected to the cloud, and who are surveilled and controlled by artificial intelligence. That's why he says nobody will have any form of privacy anymore, yet they will be 'happy'. How well Schwab masters the skill of deception with cleverly chosen words to hide his true intents, is seen at the end of his book:

'In the end, it all comes down to people and values. We need to shape a future that works for all of us by putting people first and empowering them. In its most pessimistic, dehumanized form, the 'Fourth Industrial Revolution' may indeed have the potential to "robotize" humanity and thus to deprive us of our heart and soul. But as a complement to the best parts of human nature—creativity, empathy, stewardship—it can also lift humanity into a new collective and moral consciousness based on a shared sense of destiny. It is incumbent on us all to make sure the latter prevails.' **[Then why is WEF involved in global depopulation through "vaccines"?]**

What he says here is that humans need to be empowered and may not be turned into robots, that have lost their soul. He however goes on to explain the true goal: 'lift humanity into a new collective and moral consciousness.' What does that mean? It means exactly what it says: every human will think and feel the same way, we will all share the same 'collective consciousness'.

This means total brain manipulation of all of humanity. Everyone will be submitted to the narrative that the world leaders prescribe. Humanity will have a new collective consciousness.

No longer will Google, Facebook, or Twitter need to censor anybody's voice because the Fourth Industrial Revolution will ensure that all of humanity is **'lifted into the same mindset'**. That's the ultimate goal of these criminals. The hypocrisy of Schwab is sickening, as this is exactly what he says should not happen. This is turning humans into robots who can no longer think for themselves, but who will all be forced to share the same 'mind'.

This is dealt with in detail in Chapter 14.

'The World Council for Health'
Dr Altman's Report

The very poor efficacy of these "vaccines" and the damage they cause is also thoroughly supported by Dr Altman's Report under 'The World Council for Health', where Dr Altman's conclusions are:

Ref: https://worldcouncilforhealth.org/wp-content/uploads/2022/08/Altman-Report-Final-Version-11-8-22.pdf

Conclusion

'The introduction and worldwide use of "COVID-19" gene-based 'vaccines' has been associated, in the short term, **with far more deaths, illnesses, injuries, and disabilities**

than any other therapeutic agent in the history of medicine. Due to the total lack of any long-term safety data, the potential future iatrogenic effects (including neurological, immunological and carcinogenic effects) may be even more devastating. Despite initial claims, the "COVID-19" gene-based **"vaccines"** have now been shown to possess disappointing clinical efficacy - they **neither prevent "SARS-CoV-2" infection nor do they prevent transmission of the "virus"**; any immunological protection wanes rapidly and, coincident with the emergence of the Omicron variant, **evidence of negative vaccine efficacy is being reported in many countries** including Australia. **In light of widely reported emerging and compelling evidence, there appears to be little scientific or clinical justification to support "vaccine" mandates as a health policy.'**

'The latest hospital admission statistics do not support the claim that unvaccinated individuals are more at risk of serious "COVID-19" disease, hospitalisation or death. Excess non-"COVID-19" related deaths coincident with the introduction of the gene based "vaccines" are now being reported by many countries, and **suggest a surge in heart attack and stroke among both the young, adolescents and middle-aged individuals** (especially males). Advocating the worldwide use of a new class of serious "COVID-19" gene-based "vaccines" never before deployed and advocated for use in healthy individuals of all ages regardless of clinical status (eg. natural immunity, pregnancy etc), with relatively little short-term safety data and no long-term safety data, is neither prudent or necessary and **defies the Precautionary Principle.**'

'The knowledge that the synthetic mRNA in both the **Pfizer and Moderna "vaccines" can enter the nucleus of human liver cells in culture**, raises the serious questions about genotoxicity and carcinogenicity, and adverse impact on future generations. **Disturbing safety signals regarding fertility and miscarriages are emerging.** Given the statistically or virtually nil risk of serious "COVID-19" in general affecting children aged 6 months to 11 or 12 years of age and the **clear and significant risk of serious adverse effects including myocarditis, pericarditis and death** in this age group – there seems to be little benefit to be gained by "vaccinating" these children.'

'Considerable scientific, clinical and statistical epidemiological data and understanding has been acquired since the introduction (on a provisional basis only) of the investigational "COVID-19" gene-based "vaccines". **Many of the initial ambitious claims and assumed perceptions regarding the safety and efficacy of these serious therapeutics have now been invalidated and it is now time to review and reconsider the utility of these ["vaccine"] products in light of the known unprecedented level of serious adverse reactions and death attributed to their use.'**

'The urgency for this review cannot be overestimated given the current and potential future impact on the health and wellbeing of all Australians' [and the rest of the world's population]

Dr. Phillip M. Altman

Dr. Russell Blaylock: How Vaccine-Induced Spike Proteins Damage the Brain and Cause Cancer 22nd November 2022

Retired American neurosurgeon Russell Blaylock appeared on Children's Health Defense's 'Doctors & Scientists' for an in-depth presentation about the effects of spike proteins on the body. He shared shocking discoveries about neurological damage, cancer rates, cardiac arrest and other exacerbating health issues as well as their connection to mRNA technology.

His presentation titled ***'Spike Proteins and Neurodegeneration: Effect of artificial exosomes on the nervous system in the form of an injection'*** covers the damage the spike protein does to the brain, the elderly and unborn children. He explained in detail the mechanisms that cause the damage and used several published papers to demonstrate the harm. He ends with some advice for those who have been "vaccine" injured.

Ref: https://expose-news.com/2022/11/22/how-spike-proteins-damage-brain-cause-cancer/?cmid=539a2a32-35b3-465d-a4a3-4c0b000fbd9d

Furthermore, we have this excellent and very visceral film promoted by Stew Peters,

Stew Peters Network is proud to present **WORLD PREMIERE 'DIED SUDDENLY',**

By award winning filmmakers, Matthew Skow and Nicholas Stumphauzer.

"COVID" "VACCINES"

A WORLD EXCLUSIVE SHOCKING VIDEO REPORT ON SUDDEN DEATHS AND FIBROUS CLOTS IN VEINS DUE TO "COVID" "VACCINES" Nov. 2022

THE GLOBAL "ELITE" - Why do we never believe them? For centuries, the global "elite" have broadcast their intentions to **depopulate the world** - even to the point of carving them into stone. And yet... we never seem to believe them.

Ref: https://www.covid19compensation2022.com/HOT-NEWS (click on image of fibrous clot to watch video)

Serious Side Effects Exceed the Risk of Hospitalization with COVID-19 in the Swedish Population

A recent review of phase III randomized trials of COVID-19 mRNA vaccines showed an increased risk of hospitalization for the vaccinated compared to controls. Data from the Swedish Medical Products Agency (LV) confirms that COVID-19 vaccines have resulted in a distinct increase in reported side effects, including suspected serious side effects (SSSEs) and deaths. Despite this, the consistent message from the Swedish Public Health Agency (FoHM) is that benefit outweighs risk. Does the evidence support this assertion?

With the aim of determining the relative risk of experiencing a SSSE including death, versus becoming hospitalized or dying with COVID-19, we analyzed publicly available data from LV, FoHM, the Swedish National Board of Health and Welfare (SoS) and Statistics Sweden (SCB). Assuming that 5% of all SSSEs are reported in Sweden, our analysis shows that

COVID-19 vaccination is likely to benefit one single group only – men aged over 90 years. For all other groups, the incidence of SSSEs exceeded the risk of hospitalization and death with COVID-19.

Ref: https://brownstone.org/articles/serious-side-effects-exceed-the-risk-of-hospitalization-with-covid-19-in-the-swedish-population/

USA VAERS System Reports of 31,961 cases in USA of Death from "Covid19" "vaccines"

Ref: https://www.medalerts.org/vaersdb/findfield.php?EVENTS=on&PAGENO=1&PERPAGE=10&ESORT&REVERSESORT&VAX=%28COVID19%29&VAXTYPES=%28COVID-19%29&DIED=Yes&fbclid=IwAR2rBWzmzUUh-5eWc3N4gp6PV3aEnplyzAX0Oazu32g8hzrPHqKfVmflV1M

UPDATED: How Many People Are the Vaccines Killing? – REPORT

Almost 40,000 USA deaths from vaccines reported.

Ref: **https://vernoncoleman.org/articles/how-many-people-are-vaccines-killing**

Funeral Director in UK

Dreadful Effects of "Vaccines" causing Fibrous Blood Clots

The funeral director and embalmer John O'Looney of Milton Keynes has risked his life to inform the public of the horrible fibrous blood clots caused the use of these dreadful "Covid" "vaccines", as shown in the Stew Peters video referenced above.

John O'Looney funeral director and embalmer, Quote:

'I am dealing with murder victims.'

Ref: https://www.bitchute.com/video/gigUyK3yLtMU/

CHAPTER 8

CONFIDENCE TRICK 8: PCR TESTS WORKED – THEY DID NOT

Dr. Kary Mullis, Nobel Prize winner, inventor of the PCR Test in/around 1987/1988

Quote:

'It **[PCR test]** *does not tell you if you are sick'*

Ref: Appendix I – p23 PDF Download File

One of the key strategies of the 'globalists' i.e. Evil300 is to set up public 'world' organizations, which are their visible platforms to strive to deliver their agenda. One of these has become very prominent during this organized "pandemic" and is called the World Health Organization 'WHO', which is mostly financed by **Bill Gates, a key puppet of the 'globalist' Evil300 network**. The WHO, an non-elected globalist organisation running rough shod over sovereign governments is dictating to all of humanity (- think about this!) - what we can or cannot do when it comes to our health and our own bodies.

Nobody elected the World Health Organization, and nobody wants them to be around, to bully every physician, nurse, and health practitioner into blind obedience.

The WHO forces the entire world into unquestioning submission to their dubious 'guidelines', that are more often anti-scientific than based on true science.

The WHO for example told the entire world to use the PCR test to discover "Covid" cases, while this test cannot discern between different types of pathogens and produces up to 93% of false positives. This flawed test is the main tool to tell the world there is a "pandemic", while **no medical device in history has ever been so unreliable**. Yet this anti-scientific protocol is imposed on the entire world, to promote the illusion of a global "pandemic", which is mainly based on false positives. The hundreds of millions of so-called 'Covid cases' are nothing but false positives, resulting from a fatally flawed test. **The actual "virus" "Sars-Cov-2" has never been isolated and purified, therefore it is impossible to test for it. It's a scam of astronomical proportions.**

Global PCR Test by Drosten/Corman Essentially Scientifically Worthless

An external peer review by 22 Researchers of the **Drosten/Corman** RTPCR (based upon the original test created by Kary Mullis in 1987/1988) test to detect "SARS-CoV-2" reveals **10 major scientific flaws at the molecular and methodological level** - consequences for [more than 90%] false positive results.

Ref: https://stopworldcontrol.com/downloads/science/review-drosten.pdf

The 22 Researchers:

Pieter Borger, Bobby Rajesh Malhotra, Michael Yeadon, Clare Craig, Kevin McKernan, Klaus Steger, Paul McSheehy, Lidiya Angelova, Fabio Franchi, Thomas Binder, Henrik Ullrich, Makoto Ohashi, Stefano Scoglio, Marjolein Doesburg-van Kleffens, Dorothea Gilbert, Rainer Klement, Ruth Schruefer, Berber W. Pieksma, Jan Bonte, Bruno H. Dalle Carbonare, Kevin P. Corbett, Ulrike Kämmerer.

The paper showed numerous serious flaws in the Corman-Drosten paper, the significance of which has led to **worldwide misdiagnosis of infections** attributed to "SARS-CoV-2" and associated with the disease "COVID-19".

We are confronted with stringent lockdowns which have destroyed many people's lives and livelihoods, limited access to education and these imposed restrictions by governments around the world are a direct attack on people's basic rights and their personal freedoms, resulting in collateral damage for entire economies on a global scale.

The first and major issue is that the "novel" "Coronavirus SARS-CoV-2" (in the publication named "2019-nCoV" and in February 2020 named "SARS-CoV-2" by an international consortium of virus experts) is based on in silico (theoretical) sequences, supplied by a laboratory in China, because at the time neither control material of infectious ("live") or inactivated "SARS-CoV-2" nor isolated genomic RNA of the virus was available to the authors. **To date no validation has been performed by the authorship based on isolated "SARS-CoV-2" "viruses" or full-length RNA thereof.**

The focus here should be placed upon the two stated aims: a) development and b) deployment of a diagnostic test for use in public health laboratory settings. **These aims are not achievable without having any actual virus material available** (e.g. for determining the infectious viral load).

[Corman-Drosten had NO actual virus material available – perhaps the scientific term for this is "pissing in the wind?!"] [One might question the legality of such procedures]

In any case, only a protocol with maximal accuracy can be the mandatory and primary goal in any scenario-outcome of this magnitude. Critical viral load determination is mandatory information, and it is in Christian Drosten's group responsibility to perform these experiments and provide the crucial data.

In the publication entitled ***'Detection of 2019 novel coronavirus (2019-nCoV) by real-time RT-PCR'*** (Eurosurveillance 25(8) 2020) the authors present a diagnostic workflow and RT-qPCR protocol for detection and diagnostics of "2019-nCoV" (now known as "SARS-CoV-2"), which they claim to be validated, as well as being a robust diagnostic methodology for use in public-health laboratory settings. In light of all the consequences resulting from this very publication for societies worldwide, a group of independent researchers performed a point-by-point review of the aforesaid publication in which 1) all components of the presented test design were cross checked, 2) the RT-qPCR protocol-recommendations were assessed with respect to good laboratory practice, and 3) parameters examined against relevant scientific literature covering the field.

The published RT-qPCR protocol [above] for detection and diagnostics of 2019-nCoV and the manuscript suffer from numerous technical and scientific errors, including insufficient primer design, a problematic and insufficient RT-qPCR protocol, and the absence of an accurate test validation.

Neither the presented test nor the manuscript itself fulfils the requirements for an acceptable scientific publication.

Further, **serious conflicts of interest of the authors are not mentioned.**

Finally, the very short timescale between submission and acceptance of the publication (24 hours!!!) [yes, you read it correctly 24hours!!!] signifies that a systematic peer review process was either not performed here, or of problematic [extremely] poor quality. "24 Hours" – sounds like the title of a horror film – a horror this "scientific" work certainly was!

[The time it takes for a journal to get the peer review process completed varies across journals and fields of investigation. While **some take a** month **or two, others can take up to 6 months or more, not 24 hours!]**

[The so-called peer review process of this publication, a total of 24 hours, considering the global impact of "Covid19" 90%+ false positives from the inappropriate **Drosten/Corman** RTPCR test to detect "SARS-CoV-2" should be subjected to a full investigation to ensure due diligence to obviate any possibility of civil or criminal fraud or other offences by the authors and/or those organisations supporting them in this endeavour.]

The Report by the 22 researchers into the validity of the **Drosten/Corman** Test provides compelling evidence of several scientific inadequacies, errors and flaws. For the full Report:

Ref: https://stopworldcontrol.com/downloads/science/review-drosten.pdf

The Risk of "Covid19" was Purposely Inflated by use of Inappropriate PCR Tests

The World Health Organisation 'WHO' needed "cases" in order to (unlawfully?) declare a Public Health Emergency of International Concern 'PHEIC' (so that they could announce a global "pandemic") employed a never before used Drosten-PCR test. Yet, contagion can never be detected by PCR because the test has very high incidences of false positives.

Ref: The Grand Jury Day 3 February 13 2022
Ref: https://odysee.com/@GrandJury:f/Grand-Jury-Day-3-en-online:7 hrs:mins:sec 01:51:46 to 02:09:20, Dr. Sona Pekova, Molecular Biologist, Czech Republic ***and*** hrs:min:sec 01:11:00 to 01:17:48, Prof. Dr. Ulrike Kammerer, Virologist & Immunologist, Germany

This is because the test is run on cycle thresholds (CTs) (Amplifications) and for "Covd19" they were run at well above the recommended rate (in the UK NHS run at over 40 CTs versus 25 recommended **maximum**) and using three markers in the body (subsequently reduced to two) were used to give an impression of 'rising covid19 infections' to the public.

Ref: The Grand Jury Day 3 February 13, 2022
Ref: https://odysee.com/@GrandJury:f/Grand-Jury-Day-3-en-online:7 Dr. Astrid Stuckelberger, International Health Scientist and Researcher, Switzerland min:secs 8:10 to 15:20

In order for a test to truly detect "SARS Cov-2" many different assays needed to be able to catch all the individual strains of virus. However, Drosten designed PCR in a complicated way, so as to make it applicable to anything therefore creating many false positives. The task was not to make a PCR test that was specific, but a test to produce "Covid19" "case" numbers.

Covid *Deaths* were over-counted worldwide based on the PCR Test

We are led to believe that "millions" have died **'*of* Covid'** – millions worldwide die every year. Yet all Covid deaths, anywhere, are based "on a death within 28 days of a positive (PCR) test". Whilst the average age of death – *with co-morbidities i.e., underlying conditions* – was **84** (deaths after the roll-out of the "jabs" cannot be divorced from the effects of the "jabs") the average **age of death in normal times is 82.5** i.e., the majority of those dying of "Covid" were/are ***older*** than the average age of natural death **by 1.5 years**!

Dr. Mike Yeadon *quote:*

"The PCR test is the central operational deceit"

The PCR Test is Unfit for Purpose and Never Intended for Diagnosis

The Cormen-Drosten test was a test invented by Dr. Kary Mullis, Nobel Prize winner in/around 1987/1988 that was never intended for diagnosis of illness – viral or otherwise. It was purely an amplification tool for the study of DNA and other microbiological practices. It is essentially an amplification tool, and each cycle of the test amplifies the test sample by a factor of two times. **The Test cannot diagnose ANYTHING – that is not its purpose.**

Ref 1: https://twitter.com/search?q=dr%20karry%20mullis%20pcr&src=typed_query

Ref 2: https://twitter.com/search?q=karry%20mullis&src=typed_query

Commonly known as the PCR, the Corman-Drosten test was proposed by Professor Drosten who had his own financial interest in the test to the WHO in 2020, as a mechanism that would produce "positive" — results. The worldwide testing of healthy people has grossly inflated the number of "*cases*" which, even without symptoms, were used as the basis to declare "*infections*" and, more sinisterly, to designate *deaths* ("within 28 days of a positive test") – a narrative that was constantly inflated by false mass-media causing worldwide panic.

But the **<u>Corman-Drosten protocol is entirely unscientific</u>** as asserted by Professor. Dr.Ulrike Kammerer who states in her evidence to The Grand Jury that:

"the test is so poorly designed, that it must have been intentional. Drosten who was co-author of the test, knew that if <u>used with inadequate constraint on amplification</u> the test would give positive results when people were neither sick nor infectious."

Ref: **The Grand Jury Day 1 Opening Statements – Feb 5 2022**

Ref: https://odysee.com/@GrandJury:f/Grand-Jury-1-EN:0 – mins:secs 38:08 to 46:14,

N.Ana Garner, Attorney at Law, USA)

'The basis of the [Covid19] "pandemic" was a big lie...a criminal collaboration... irrefutable evidence of fraud and malfeasance...'

The PCR was and is run at cycles way above the recommended Cycle Threshold (CT) ***<u>including by the UK NHS</u>***

Information given by the US Center of Diseases Control (CDC) and US Federal Drug Administration (FDA) is demonstrably false and the **Grand Jury has evidence that Drosten knew the test was meaningless and false**. The WHO recommended grossly excessive cycle thresholds, far beyond industry standards, which rendered any test meaningless. **False positive rates of PCR are close to 97%.**

PCR tests have been used to drive "Covid19" figures higher than what they really were. The false tests have caused huge catastrophic harm to the populace of the world. There is irrefutable evidence of fraud and malfeasance throughout the Covid19 practice regime.
Ref: The Grand Jury Day 3 – Feb 13 2022
Ref: https://odysee.com/@GrandJury:f/Grand-Jury-Day-3-en-online:7 mins:secs 15:00 to 21:47, Dr. Astrid Stuckelberger, Former WHO adviser and International Health Scientist) see below:

In January 2020, the US Centers for Disease Control and Prevention CDC warned that the <u>PCR did not work, it was not designed to monitor an epidemic nor to validate an infectious disease.</u> WHO (World Health Organisation) alerted that the PCR test should be looked at with caution, this was hidden on the WHO website. WHO said every country which used PCR test should write down clearly the amplification cycle with the result.

The WHO was never a seller of "vaccines" or medications. The way PCR test applied needs discussion -why is it inserted so deeply into the nose, near the sensitive pre brain, which is not necessary; this PCR test can "vaccinate" people, as done by vets. This invasive procedure should be subjected to full independent scrutiny.

The PCR test has enabled the lie of asymptomatic transmission.

Note: For "asymptomatic" read "not showing any relevant symptoms"

'This **[asymptomatic/not showing any relevant symptoms]** ***is the central conceptual deceit.***

If true, then anyone might infect and kill you. Falsely claimed asymptomatic transmission underscores **[permits]** ***almost every intrusion: masking, mass testing, lockdowns, border restrictions, school closures, even vaccine passports'***

Ref: Dr Mike Yeadon ***'The Covid Lies'***

CHAPTER 9

CONFIDENCE TRICK 9: FACIAL MASKS WORKED – THEY DID NOT

Dr. Heiko Schoening - German Corona Investigation Committee

Quote:

'You may as well throw sand at a **[fishing]** *net as wear a mask to catch a "virus"'*

Ref: Appendix I – p27 PDF Download File

The Stanford [Covid19] Mask Study
Baruch Vainshelboim
This report carries 67 independent citations

Ref: https://stopworldcontrol.com/downloads/science/Stanford-Mask-Study.pdf

Many countries across the globe utilized medical and non-medical facemasks as non-pharmaceutical intervention for reducing the transmission and infectivity of "coronavirus disease-2019" ("COVID-19"). Although, scientific evidence supporting facemasks' efficacy is lacking, adverse physiological, psychological and health effects are established. Is has been hypothesized that facemasks have compromised safety and efficacy profile and should be avoided from use. The current article comprehensively summarizes scientific evidence with respect to wearing facemasks in the "COVID-19" era, providing proper research-based data and information for public health and decisions making.

Breathing Physiology

Breathing is one of the most important physiological functions to sustain life and health. The Human body requires a continuous and adequate oxygen (O2) supply to all organs and cells for normal functioning and survival. Breathing is also an essential process for removing metabolic by-products [carbon dioxide (CO2)] occurring during cell respiration. It is well established that acute significant deficit in O2 (hypoxemia) and increased levels of CO2 (hypercapnia) even for few minutes can be severely harmful and lethal, while chronic hypoxemia and hypercapnia cause health deterioration, exacerbation of existing conditions, morbidity and ultimately mortality.

Emergency medicine demonstrates that 5–6 min of severe hypoxemia during cardiac arrest will cause brain death with extremely poor survival rates.

Efficacy of Face Masks – [None – Essentially Useless and Harmful]

The physical properties of medical and non-medical facemasks suggest that facemasks are **ineffective to block viral particles due to their difference in scales**. According to the current knowledge, the "virus" "SARS-CoV-2" **has a diameter of 60 nm to 140 nm** [nanometers (billionth of a meter)], while **medical and non-medical facemasks' thread diameter ranges from 55 μm to 440 μm** [micrometers (one millionth of a meter), **which is more than 1000 times larger than the "Sars-Cov2" virus diameter.**

[Although these people responsible for this nightmare – Bill Gates, Anthony Fauci, World Health Organisation 'WHO' Director-General, Dr. Tedros Adhanom Ghebreyesus, World Economic Forum WEF, Chairman, Klaus Schwab, the 'Thirteen Families', Evil300 etc may be intellectual 'garden gnomes' as well as moral 'garden gnomes', it does not take the intellect of Johann Wolfgang von Goethe to work out the following:]

Due to the difference in sizes between "SARS-CoV-2" diameter and facemasks thread diameter (the virus is 1000 times smaller), "SARS-CoV-2" can easily pass through any facemask.

It is clear that "Covid19" 'Face masks' had nothing to do with health. They were imposed upon the global population as a means of inflicting fear and loss of identity throughout the world.

[They also were very likely to cause harm since they restricted the flow of oxygen to the body and brain and increased the flow of carbon dioxide, which is a human effluent, to the body and brain. The mask wearers were breathing his/her own carbon dioxide effluent into the mask and then breathing it back in to his/her lungs!]

[This is rather like encouraging the global population to eat their own physical effluent i.e., faeces!]

In addition, the efficiency filtration rate of facemasks is poor, ranging from 0.7% in non-surgical, cotton gauze woven mask to 26% in cotton material. With respect to surgical and N95 medical facemasks, the efficiency filtration rate falls to 15% and 58%, respectively when even a small gap between the mask and the face exists.

Clinical scientific evidence challenges further the efficacy of facemasks to block human-to-human transmission or infectivity. A randomised controlled trial (RCT) of 246 participants [123 (50%) symptomatic)] who were allocated to either wearing or not wearing surgical facemask, assessing viruses' transmission including coronavirus. **The results of this study showed that among symptomatic individuals (those with fever, cough, sore throat, runny nose etc...) there was no difference between wearing and not wearing facemask for coronavirus droplets transmission of particles of >5 μm.**

Among asymptomatic [having no "Covid19" symptoms] individuals, there was no droplets or aerosols coronavirus detected from any participant with or without the mask, **suggesting that asymptomatic [having no "Covid19" symptoms] individuals do not transmit or infect other people. [Is this because they do not have "Covid19"? – Might explain it!]**

This was further supported by a study on infectivity where 445 asymptomatic individuals were exposed to a symptomatic "SARS-CoV2" carrier (been positive for "SARS-CoV2") using close contact (shared quarantine space) for a median of 4 to 5 days. **The study found that NONE of the 445 individuals was infected with "SARS-CoV-2".**

A meta-analysis among health care workers found that compared to no masks, surgical mask and N95 respirators were not effective against transmission of viral infections or influenza-like illness based on six RCTs [Randomised Control Trials]. Using separate analysis of 23 observational studies, this meta-analysis **found no protective effect of medical mask or N95 respirators against "SARS2" "virus".** A recent systematic review of 39 studies including 33,867 participants in community settings (self-report illness), found no difference between N95 respirators versus surgical masks and surgical mask versus no masks in the risk for developing influenza or influenza-like illness, **suggesting their <u>ineffectiveness of blocking viral transmissions</u> in community settings.**

World Health Organisation 'WHO' Makes it Up as it Goes Along!

In an early publication the WHO stated that **'facemasks are not required, as no evidence is available on its usefulness to protect non-sick persons'**. In the same publication, the WHO declared that **'cloth (e. g. cotton or gauze) masks are not recommended under any circumstance'. Conversely, in later publication the WHO stated** that the usage of fabric-made facemasks (Polypropylene, Cotton, Polyester, Cellulose, Gauze and Silk) is a general community practice for 'preventing the infected wearer transmitting the virus to others and/or to offer protection to the healthy wearer against infection (prevention)'. **The same publication further conflicted itself** by stating that due to the lower filtration, breathability and overall performance of fabric facemasks, the usage of woven fabric mask such as cloth, and/or nonwoven fabrics, should only be considered for infected persons and not for prevention practice in asymptomatic individuals.

Physiological effects of wearing facemasks – [Harmful]

Wearing facemask mechanically restricts breathing by increasing the resistance of air movement during both inhalation and exhalation process. Although, intermittent (several times a week) and repetitive (10–15 breaths for 2–4 sets) increase in respiration resistance may be adaptive for strengthening respiratory muscles, **<u>prolonged and continuous effect of wearing facemask is maladaptive and could be detrimental for health</u>.**

In addition to hypoxia and hypercapnia, breathing through facemask residues bacterial and germs components on the inner and outside layer of the facemask. These toxic components are repeatedly rebreathed back into the body, causing self-contamination. Breathing through facemasks also increases temperature and humidity in the space between the mouth and the mask, resulting **a release of toxic particles from the mask's materials. A systematic literature review estimated that aerosol contamination levels of facemasks [was significant] including 13 to 202,549 different viruses.** Rebreathing contaminated air with high bacterial and toxic particle concentrations along with low O2 and high CO2 levels continuously challenge the body homeostasis, causing self-toxicity and immunosuppression.

A study among 158 health-care workers using protective personal equipment primarily N95 facemasks reported that 81% (128 workers) developed new headaches during their work shifts as these become **mandatory** due to "COVID-19" outbreak. For those who used the N95 facemask greater than 4 h per day, the likelihood for developing a headache during the work shift was approximately four times higher [Odds ratio = 3.91, 95% CI (1.35–11.31) p = 0.012], while 82.2% of the N95 wearers developed the headache already within ≤10 to 50 minutes.

Psychological effects of wearing facemasks - Harmful

Psychologically, wearing facemask fundamentally has negative effects on the wearer and the nearby person. **Basic human-to-human connectivity through face expression is compromised and self-identity is somewhat eliminated.** These dehumanizing movements partially delete the uniqueness and individuality of person who wearing the facemask as well as the connected person. **Social connections and relationships are basic human needs, which are innately inherited in all people, whereas reduced human-to-human connections are associated with poor mental and physical health.**

A meta-analysis of 91 studies of about 400,000 people showed a 13% increased mortality risk among people with low contact to high contact frequency. Another meta-analysis of 148 prospective studies (308,849 participants) found that poor social relationships were associated with 50% increased mortality risk. **People who were socially isolated or felt lonely had 45% and 40% increased mortality risk, respectively**. These findings were consistent across ages, sex, initial health status, cause of death and follow-up periods.

[Face masks as prescribed for "Covid19" are likely to encourage low frequency of contact among people.]

Conclusions

The existing scientific evidence challenge the safety and efficacy of wearing facemasks as preventive intervention for "COVID-19". **The data suggest that both medical and non-medical facemasks are ineffective to block human-to-human transmission of viral and infectious disease such "SARS-CoV2" and "COVID-19", supporting against the usage of facemasks.**

Wearing facemasks has been demonstrated to have substantial adverse physiological and psychological effects. These include hypoxia, hypercapnia, shortness of breath, increased acidity and toxicity, activation of fear and stress response, rise in stress hormones, immunosuppression, fatigue, headaches, decline in cognitive performance, predisposition for viral and infectious illnesses, chronic stress, anxiety, and depression. Long-term consequences of wearing facemask can cause health deterioration, developing and progression of chronic diseases and premature death.

Governments, policy makers and health organizations should utilize proper and scientific evidence-based approach with respect to wearing facemasks, when the latter is considered as preventive intervention for public health.

This Report is supported by many similar research papers:

Masks Don't Work A review of science relevant to COVID-19 social policy
Denis G. Rancourt, PhD

Ref: https://stopworldcontrol.com/downloads/en/legal/science/rancourt.pdf

Summary / Abstract

Masks and respirators do not work.

There have been extensive randomised controlled trial (RCT) studies, and meta-analysis reviews of RCT studies, which all show that masks and respirators do not work to prevent respiratory influenza-like illnesses, or respiratory illnesses believed to be transmitted by droplets and aerosol particles. Furthermore, the relevant known physics and biology, which Dr. Rancourt reviewed, are such that masks and respirators should not work. It would be a paradox if masks and respirators worked, given what we know about viral respiratory diseases: **The main transmission path is long-residence-time aerosol particles (< 2.5 μm), which are too fine to be blocked**, and the minimum-infective-dose is smaller than one aerosol particle.

The present paper about masks illustrates the degree to which governments, the mainstream media, and institutional propagandists can decide to operate in a science vacuum or select only incomplete science that serves their interests. Such recklessness is also certainly the case with the current global [Covid19] lockdown of over 1 billion people, an unprecedented experiment in medical and political history.

The is *no* evidence that masks work against "Sars-Cov-22"/" Covid19"

The Brownstone Institute is a nonprofit 501(c)(3) organization founded May 2021 has collated over 150 studies into the ineffectiveness of masks and their harm in their use in the "Covid19" mandates: - December 2021
by
Paul Elias Alexander

Ref: https://brownstone.org/articles/more-than-150-comparative-studies-and-articles-on-mask-ineffectiveness-and-harms/

Introduction

It is not unreasonable to conclude that surgical and cloth masks, used as they currently are being used (without other forms of PPE protection), have no impact on controlling the transmission of "Covid-19" virus. Current evidence implies that face masks can be actually harmful.

The body of evidence indicates that face masks are largely ineffective.

The focus of this Report is on "COVID" face masks and the prevailing science that we have had for nearly 20 months.

The Report builds on the fine work done by Gupta, Kulldorff, and Bhattacharya on the **Great Barrington Declaration (GBD)** and similar impetus by Dr. Scott Atlas.

Because we saw very early on that the lockdowns were the single greatest mistake in public health history. **We knew the history and knew they would not work**. We also knew very early of "COVID's" risk stratification.

Sadly, our children will bear the catastrophic consequences and not just educationally, of the deeply flawed school closure policy for decades to come (particularly our minority children who were least able to afford this).

Many are still pressured to wear masks and punished for not doing so.

The Report presents the masking 'body of evidence' below (n=167 studies and pieces of evidence), comprised of comparative effectiveness research as well as related evidence and high-level reporting.

To date, the evidence has been stable and clear that masks do not work to control the "virus" and they can be harmful and especially to children.

Ref: https://brownstone.org/articles/more-than-150-comparative-studies-and-articles-on-mask-ineffectiveness-and-harms/

CHAPTER 10

CONFIDENCE TRICK 10: LOCKDOWNS WORKED – THEY DID NOT

Dr. Mike Yeadon former Vice President, Head of Respiratory Health, Pfizer Pharmaceuticals (UK)

Quote:

'They* [lockdowns] *most certainly - as has been seen consequently (particularly in comparative data from Sweden which had no formal lockdown) - did not slow down the spread or reduce the number of* [Covid19] *cases and deaths.'

Ref: Appendix I – p31 PDF Download File

Dr Richard Fleming PhD, MD, JD Distinguished Physician & Doctor of Law USA, Author:

'Is Covid-19 a Bioweapon? A Scientific and Forensic Investigation' – The Interview

["Covid19" is more likely perhaps, on the evidence, to be a Chemical Weapon rather than a Bioweapon]

Ref: https://australiaoneparty.com/truth-about-covid-coming-out-now/
for all Dr Richard Fleming quotations.

Dr Richard Fleming quote:

'We took procedures in 2020 and 2021 that made no scientific sense. There is no data to show that the quarantining of citizens around the world stopped the "virus". The authorities violated the International Covenant on Civil and Political Rights. They have violated the American Medical Association Code of Ethics.'

'Physicians abandoned the practice of medicine for a variety of reasons; many of them did so because they were told there were no treatments.' [which there were – see Chapter 15]

'Who told them that there were no alternative working treatments?'

'All the things that we used to do in medicine; in 2020, 2021, 2022 were thrown out the window.'

'We locked down society.' 'We put fear into everybody's heart.'

'We told people to quit believing people who might tell you something different.'

'We quit challenging the "scientific" paradigm and free exchange of medical ideas has not been done.'

There were not just physical lockdowns; there were psychological, information flow, freedom of expression and movement lockdowns.

Assessing Mandatory Stay-at-home and Business Closure Effects on the spread of "Covid19"

by

Eran Bendavid, Christopher Oh, Jay Bhattacharya, John P.A. Ioannidis

Departments:

Department of Medicine, Stanford University Stanford, CA
Center for Health Policy and the Center for Primary Care and Outcomes Research, Stanford University, Stanford, CA
Department of Epidemiology and Population Health, Stanford University, Stanford, CA
Department of Biomedical Data Science, Stanford University, Stanford, CA Department of Statistics, Stanford University, Stanford, CA 6Meta-Research Innovation Center at Stanford (METRICS), Stanford University, Stanford, CA

Note: Prof. John P.A. Ioannidis is the most cited expert in the world in his field.

Ref: https://stopworldcontrol.com/downloads/science/lockdowns-paper.pdf

Introduction

The spread of "COVID-19" has led to multiple policy responses that aim to reduce the transmission of the "SARS-CoV-2". The principal goal of these so-called non-pharmaceutical interventions (NPIs) is to reduce transmission in the absence of pharmaceutical options in order to reduce resultant death, disease, and health system overload. Some of the most restrictive NPI policies include mandatory stay-at-home and business closure orders ("lockdowns"). The early adoption of these more restrictive non-pharmaceutical interventions (mrNPIs) in early 2020 was justified because of the "rapid spread of the "disease"", "overwhelmed health systems in some hard-hit places", and "substantial uncertainty about the "virus" morbidity and mortality". Because of the potential harmful health effects of mrNPI – including hunger, opioid-related overdoses, missed vaccinations, increase in non-"COVID" "diseases" from missed health services, domestic abuse, mental health and suicidality, as well as a host of economic consequences with health implications – it is increasingly recognized that their postulated benefits deserve careful study.

Background and Aims

The most restrictive non-pharmaceutical interventions (NPIs) for controlling the spread of COVID-19 **are mandatory stay-at-home and business closures**. Given the consequences of these policies, it is important to assess their effects. We evaluate the effects on epidemic case growth of more restrictive NPIs (mrNPIs), above and beyond those of less restrictive NPIs (lrNPIs).

Methods

We first estimate "COVID-19" case growth in relation to any NPI implementation in subnational regions of 10 countries: England, France, Germany, Iran, Italy, Netherlands, Spain, South Korea, Sweden, and the US. Using first-difference models with fixed effects, we isolate the effects of mrNPIs by subtracting the combined effects of lrNPIs and epidemic dynamics from all NPIs. We use case growth in Sweden and South Korea, two countries that did not implement mandatory stay-at-home and business closures, as comparison countries for the other 8 countries (16 total comparisons).

Results

Implementing any NPIs was associated with significant reductions in case growth in 9 out of 10 studies countries; including South Korea and Sweden that implemented only lrNPIs (Spain had a non-significant effect). **After subtracting the epidemic and lrNPI effects, we find no clear, significant beneficial effect of mrNPIs on case growth in any country.** In France, e.g., the effect of mrNPIs was +7% (95CI -5%-19%) when compared with Sweden, and +13% (-12%-38%) when compared with South Korea (positive means pro-contagion). The 95% confidence intervals excluded 30% declines in all 16 comparisons and 15% declines in 11/16 comparisons.

Conclusions

While small benefits cannot be excluded, **we do not find significant benefits on case growth of more restrictive NPIs.** Similar reductions in case growth may be achievable with less restrictive interventions.

More than 500 medical doctors wrote to President Trump, warning him that lockdowns destroy the lives of millions of people

Ref: https://stopworldcontrol.com/downloads/science/letter.pdf

President Donald J. Trump
The White House
1600 Pennsylvania Avenue,
NW Washington,
D.C. 20500

May 19, 2020

Dear Mr. President:

Thousands of physicians in all specialties and from all States would like to express our gratitude for your leadership. **We write to you today to express our alarm over the exponentially growing negative health consequences of the national shutdown. In medical terms, the shutdown was a mass casualty incident.**

During a mass casualty incident, victims are immediately triaged to black, red, yellow, or green. The first group, triage level black, includes those who require too many resources to save during a mass crisis. The red group has severe injuries that are survivable with treatment, the yellow group has serious injuries that are not immediately life threatening, and the green group has minor injuries.

The red group receives highest priority. The next priority is to ensure that the other two groups do not deteriorate a level. Decades of research have shown that by strictly following this algorithm, we save the maximum number of lives.

Millions of Americans are already at triage level red. These include 150,000 Americans per month who would have had a new cancer detected through routine screening that hasn't happened, millions who have missed routine dental care to fix problems strongly linked to heart disease/death, and preventable cases of stroke, heart attack, and child abuse. **Suicide hotline phone calls have increased 600%.**

Tens of millions are at triage level yellow. **Liquor sales have increased 300-600%,** cigarettes sales have increased, **rent has gone unpaid, family relationships have become frayed, and millions of well-child check-ups have been missed.**

Hundreds of millions are at triage level green. These are people who currently are solvent, but at risk should economic conditions worsen. Poverty and financial uncertainty are closely linked to poor health.

A continued shutdown means hundreds of millions of Americans will downgrade a level. The following are real examples from our practices.

Patient E.S. is a mother with two children whose office job was reduced to part-time and whose husband was furloughed. The father is drinking more, the mother is depressed and not managing her diabetes well and the children are barely doing any schoolwork.

Patient A.F. has chronic but previously stable health conditions. Her elective hip replacement was delayed, which caused her to become nearly sedentary, resulting in a pulmonary embolism in April.

Patient R.T. is an elderly nursing home patient, who had a small stroke in early March but was expected to make a nearly complete recovery. Since the shutdown, he has had no physical or speech therapy, and no visitors. He has lost weight and is deteriorating rather than making progress.

Patient S.O. is a college freshman who cannot return to normal life, school, and friendships. He risks depression, alcohol abuse, drug abuse, trauma, and future financial uncertainty.

We are alarmed at what appears to be the lack of consideration for the future health of our patients. The downstream health effects of deteriorating a level are being massively under-estimated and under-reported. This is an order of magnitude error. [10*]

It is impossible to overstate the short, medium, and long-term harm to people's health with a continued shutdown. Losing a job is one of life's most stressful events, and the effect on a person's health is not lessened because it also has happened to 30 million other people. Keeping schools and universities closed is incalculably detrimental for children, teenagers, and young adults for decades to come.

The millions of casualties of a continued shutdown will be hiding in plain sight, but they will be called alcoholism, homelessness, suicide, heart attack, stroke, or kidney failure. In youths it will be called financial instability, unemployment, despair, drug addiction, unplanned pregnancies, poverty, and abuse.

Because the harm is diffuse, there are those who hold that it does not exist. We, the undersigned, know otherwise. Please let us know if we may be of assistance.

Respectfully,

Simone Gold, M.D., J.D. & >500 physicians (attached)

Lockdowns Do Not Control The "Coronavirus"
December 2020
By
American Institute for Economic Research

Ref: https://stopworldcontrol.com/downloads/science/lockdowns-evidence.pdf

Founded in 1933, the American Institute for Economic Research (AIER) is one of the oldest and most respected nonpartisan economic research and advocacy organizations in the country. With a global reach and influence, AIER is dedicated to developing and promoting the ideas of pure freedom and private governance by combining advanced economic research with accessible media outreach and educational programming to cultivate a better, broader understanding of the fundamental principles that enable peace and prosperity around the world.

The use of universal lockdowns in the event of the appearance of a new pathogen has no precedent. It has been a science experiment in real time, with **most of the human population used as lab rats. The costs are legion.** The question is whether lockdowns worked to control the virus in a way that is scientifically verifiable. **Based on the following studies, the answer is no and for a variety of reasons: bad data, no correlations, no causal demonstration, anomalous exceptions, and so on.**

There is no relationship between lockdowns (or whatever else people want to call them to mask their true nature) and "virus" control.

Perhaps this is a shocking revelation, given that universal social and economic controls are becoming the new orthodoxy. In a saner world, the burden of proof really should belong to the 'lock-downers', since it is they who **overthrew 100 years of public-health wisdom** and replaced it with an **untested, top-down imposition on freedom and human rights**. They never accepted that burden. **They took it as axiomatic that a "virus" could be intimidated and frightened by credentials, edicts, speeches, and masked gendarmes**.

[The editor can confidently assert that "viruses" are not capable of identifying masked gendarmes nor are they capable of understanding either their relevance or their stupidity.]

Thirty-five research papers supporting the conclusions above are then cited in the research paper.

Ref: https://stopworldcontrol.com/downloads/science/lockdowns-evidence.pdf

Harmful Effects of Lockdowns

By

America's Frontline Doctors

America's Frontline Doctors Ref: https://aflds.org/ 'AFLDS' created this overview of proven harmful effects of lockdowns on the population:

AFLDS policy statement on the harmful health effects of lockdowns.

Lockdowns are not effective, as seen by many scientific studies, common sense, and worldwide observation. Locking down entire communities was never before done in all of recorded human history, but it swept the globe in 2020. In addition to not stopping the transmission of a tiny respiratory "virus" that fortunately does not permanently harm the vast majority of people, lockdowns cause insurmountable negative health effects. These range from the worsening of chronic stable conditions, to missing new serious diagnoses, to missing necessary treatments, and very often death. And where lack of medical care and social isolation intersect, the tragedy of addiction, substance abuse, depression, trauma, and crime repeats itself in ever escalating numbers. **The death and illness due to lockdowns is exponentially higher than deaths due to "Covid-19".** This is all the more tragic because most "Covid19" deaths are at or after the average life expectancy but most of the death and illness due to lockdowns is in younger persons.

Economic Damage

1. February-April unemployment increased by 12% women and 10% men https://www.bls.gov/charts/employment-situation/civilian-unemployment-rate.htm
2. In March 39% of people living with a household income of ≤ $40,000 lost their job https://www.federalreserve.gov/publications/files/2019-report-economic-well-being-us-h ouseholds-202005.pdf [page not found]

3. 40% restaurants expect to be out of business by March 2021 [page not found] https://www.qsrmagazine.com/consumer-trends/only-45-percent-restaurants-are-confiden t-theyll-last-year and 75% independent restaurants have new debt >$50,000 https://www.fsrmagazine.com/finance/some-independent-restaurants-arent-sure-theyll-m ake-it-november [page not found]
4. The long-term unemployed, defined as those out of work for 27 weeks or more, hit its highest-ever month-to-month increase last summer. https://www.nelp.org/blog/unemployment-payments-running-millions-even-long-term-un employment-surges/ [page not found]
5. Lockdowns cause huge supply push and demand-pull global inflation

Ref: https://brownstone.org/articles/a-world-on fire/?utm_medium=onesignal&utm_source=push [page not found]

Healthcare

1. Emergency visits declined 42% from 2.1 million to 1.2 million/week CDC https://www.cdc.gov/mmwr/volumes/69/wr/mm6923e1.htm
2. Chemotherapy admissions down 45-66% and urgent cancer referrals 70-89% decrease https://www.researchgate.net/publication/340984562_Estimating_excess_mortality_in_p eople_with_cancer_and_multimorbidity_in_the_COVID-19_emergency
3. 38% decrease in serious heart attack treatments in the USA https://www.jacc.org/doi/pdf/10.1016/j.jacc.2020.04.011
4. 40% nationwide decrease in stroke cases. https://www.medscape.com/view article/930374?src=wnl_edit_tpal&uac=75658DK&imp ID=2380219&faf=1
5. 51.8% drop in breast cancer diagnosis vs. 2018 https://jamanetwork.com/journals/jamanetworkopen/fullarticle/2768946
6. Hospital financial losses $323.1 billion in 2020 https://revcycleintelligence.com/news/aha-projects-323b-in-covid-19-hospital-financial-l osses-in-2020 [page not found]

Mental Health

1. More than 40 states report increase in opioid overdose https://www.ama-assn.org/system/files/2020-11/issue-brief-increases-in-opioid-related-overdose.pdf
2. 13% more people using drugs https://www.cdc.gov/mmwr/volumes/69/wr/mm6932a1.htm
3. In New York, google searches for "anxiety, panic attack, insomnia" increased about 20% https://jamanetwork.com/journals/jamainternalmedicine/fullarticle/2771502
4. More than twice as many suicide thoughts (10.7% vs. 4.2%) and age 18-24, 25.5%, three times higher anxiety, and four times higher rates of depression. https://www.cdc.gov/mmwr/volumes/69/wr/mm6932a1.htm

Children/Youth

1. Decrease in life expectancy by 5.53 million years of life due to COVID school closures https://jamanetwork.com/journals/jamanetworkopen/fullarticle/10.1001/jamanetworkope n.2020.28786 [page not found]
2. Decrease in overall life options/choices (>30,0000 internships were lost 52%) March 9-April 13 https://www.glassdoor.com/research/internship-hiring-coronavirus/
3. Rate of food insecurity (2018-2020) has doubled from 14% to 32% for households with children https://www.brookings.edu/research/ten-facts-about-covid-19-and-the-u-s-economy/#:~:text=The%20COVID%2D19%20crisis%20also,(U.S.%20Census%20Bureau%202020a). [page not found]
4. Emergency visits for mental health for age 5-11 increased 24% and 12-17 increased 31%, year over year https://www.cdc.gov/mmwr/volumes/69/wr/mm6945a3.htm?s_cid=mm6945a3_w

Homicide

1. January-June 2020: murder and manslaughter increased nearly 15%, arson increased nearly 20% (and more than 50% in dense cities) https://www.fbi.gov/news/pressrel/press-releases/overview-of-preliminary-uniform-crime-report-january-june-2020 [page not found]
2. June-August 2020 homicides increased 53% compared to 2019 https://covid19.counciloncj.org/2020/09/26/impact-report-covid-19-and-crime/

Note: These USA figures are most likely to be similarly recorded in UK and all other countries that followed the "Covid19" 'Lockdown' false paradigm. The health 'costs' in 'Lockdowns' most probably dwarf the cost of the fatalities of "Covid19" - being 0.14%.

Some of these links give the error message 'page not found'. I will leave the reader to research why these pages are no longer available, when they were available in the initial report.

CHAPTER 11

CONFIDENCE TRICK 11: THERE WERE FEW ADVERSE EFFECTS – THERE WERE MANY

The "Vaccine" Death Report
Evidence of millions of deaths and serious adverse events resulting from the experimental "COVID-19" injections
by
Dr David John Sorenson & Dr Vladimir Zelenko

September 2021

Ref: https://stopworldcontrol.com/downloads/en/vaccines/vaccinereport.pdf

Note that the data for the Report is based primarily upon data from USA. However, the prime driver for the "pandemic" was trans-global, so the data applicable to USA is most probably applicable to many other countries in the world that were working in a perfect lockstep unison in the roll-out of the fake "pandemic".

Purpose

The purpose of this report is to document how all over the world millions of people have died, and hundreds of millions of serious adverse events have occurred, after injections with the experimental mRNA gene therapy. **We also reveal the real risk of an unprecedented genocide.**

Facts

We aim to only present scientific facts and stay away from unfounded claims. The data is clear and verifiable. Over one hundred references can be found for all presented information, which is provided as a starting point for further investigation.

Complicity

The data suggests that we may currently be witnessing the greatest organized mass murder in the history of our world. The severity of this situation compels us to ask this critical question: will we rise to the defense of billions of innocent people? Or will we permit personal profit over justice, and be complicit? Networks of lawyers all over the world are preparing class-action lawsuits to prosecute all who are serving this criminal agenda. To all who have been complicit so far, we say: There is still time to turn and choose the side of truth. Please make the right choice.

Worldwide

Although this report focuses on the situation in the United States, it also applies to the rest of the world, as the same type of experimental injections with similar death rates - and comparable systems of corruption to hide these numbers - are used worldwide. Therefore, we encourage everyone around the world to share this report. May it be a wake-up call for all of humanity.

CDC Whistle-Blower Signs Sworn Affidavit

VAERS data from the American CDC shows that as of September 17, 2021, already 726,963 people suffered adverse events, including **stroke, heart failure, blood clots, brain disorders, convulsions, seizures, inflammations of brain & spinal cord, life-threatening allergic reactions, autoimmune diseases, arthritis, miscarriage, infertility, rapid-onset muscle weakness, deafness, blindness, narcolepsy, and cataplexy**.

Besides the astronomical number of severe side effects, the CDC reports that **15,386 people died** as a result of receiving the **experimental injections**. However, a **CDC healthcare fraud detection expert named Jane Doe** investigated this and came to the shocking discovery that the number **of deaths is <u>at least five times higher</u> than what the CDC is admitting.** In fact, in her initial communications to professor in medicine Dr. Peter McCullough, this whistle blower said that the **<u>number of deaths is ten times higher</u>**. The CDC health fraud detection expert signed an affidavit, in which she stated her findings. She carefully chose the wordings *'...**under-reported by a conservative factor of at least five'***, but as she revealed initially, **the factor could also be ten**. Here is an excerpt of the affidavit:

*'I have, over the last 25 years, developed over 100 distinct healthcare fraud detection algorithms. ... When the "COVID-19"" vaccine" clearly became associated with patient death and harm, I was inclined to investigate the matter. It is my professional estimate that VAERS (the Vaccine Adverse Event Reporting System) database, while extremely useful, is **under-reported by a conservative factor of at least 5**. ... and have assessed that the **<u>deaths occurring within 3 days of vaccination are higher than those reported in VAERS by a factor of at least 5</u>**.'*

According to this CDC health fraud detection expert the **number of "vaccine" deaths in the U.S. is not 15,386 but somewhere <u>between 80,000 and 160,000</u>. These inaccuracies of such low "Covid19" figures for deaths are probably typical of most countries in the world including the UK.**

*The CDC is also **vastly underreporting other adverse events**, like severe allergic reactions (anaphylaxis). The Informed Consent Action Network (ICAN) reported that a study showed how the **<u>actual number of anaphylaxes is 50 to 120 times higher than claimed by the CDC</u>**.*

*On top of that, a private researcher took a close look at the VAERS database and tried looking up specific case-ID's. He found countless examples where **<u>the original death records were deleted,</u>** and in some cases, the numbers have been switched for milder reactions.*

*He says: **'What the analysis of all the case numbers is telling us right now is that there's approximately 150,000 cases that are missing, that were there, that are no longer there. The question is, are they all deaths?'***

Criminal Activity by CDC (USA)

How criminal the CDC is, was also revealed a few years ago, when researchers investigated the link between vaccines and autism. They found that there indeed is a direct connection. So, what did the CDC do? All the researchers came together, and a large dustbin was placed in the middle of the room. In it they threw all the documents that showed the link between autism and vaccinations. Thus, the evidence was destroyed. Subsequently, a so-called 'scientific' article was published in Pediatric, stating that vaccinations do not cause autism. However, a leading scientist within the CDC, **William Thompson, exposed this crime**. He publicly admitted*:*

'I was involved in misleading millions of people about the possible negative side effects of vaccines. We lied about the scientific findings.'

The worst example of **criminal methodology used to hide vaccine deaths** is the fact that the CDC doesn't consider a person vaccinated until two weeks after their second injection. This means that anyone who dies during the weeks before or the two weeks after the second injection, are considered unvaccinated deaths, and are therefore not counted as vaccine deaths. By doing this, they can ignore the vast majority of deaths following the injection. **This is the number 1 method used in nations worldwide to hide the countless numbers of vaccine deaths. [Including the UK.]**

Moderna Hides 300,000 Adverse Events

A whistle-blower from Moderna made a screenshot of an internal company notice labelled "Confidential - For internal distribution only", showing there were 300,000 adverse events reported in only three months:

'This enabled the team to effectively manage approximately 300,000 adverse event reports and 30,000 medical information requests in a three-month span to support the global launch of their "COVID-19" "vaccine".'

50,000 Medicare "Vaccinated" Died

Attorney Thomas Renz received information from a whistle-blower inside the Centers for Medicare & Medicaid Service (CMS), which reveals how **48,465 people died shortly after receiving their injections**. He emphasized that these death numbers are from only 18% of the U.S. population. If we apply this to **the entire U.S. population, that would mean a death rate of ± 250,000**. Other factors also play a role of course, such as the age of the Medicare patients, and the younger members of the American people, so we can't simply extrapolate this to the entire U.S. population. **But we do see that something extremely serious is going on.**

All this information already shows us that the number of adverse events and deaths is a multitude of what is being told to the public. The situation is however still far worse than most of us can even imagine. The famous Lazarus report from Harvard Pilgrim Health Care inc. in 2009 revealed that **in general only 1% of adverse events from vaccines is being reported:**

'Adverse events from drugs and vaccines are common but underreported. Although 25% of ambulatory patients experience an adverse drug event, less than 0.3% of all adverse drug events and 1-13% of serious events are reported to the Food and Drug Administration (FDA). Likewise, fewer than 1% of vaccine adverse events are reported.'

A local ABC News Station in USA posted a request on Facebook for people to share their stories of **unvaccinated loved ones that died**. They wanted to make a news story on this. What happened was totally unexpected. In five days' time over **250,000 people posted comments**, but not about unvaccinated loved ones. **All the comments talk about vaccinated loved ones that died shortly after being injected, or that are disabled for life**. The 250,000 comments reveal a shocking death wave among the population, and the heart wrenching suffering these injections are causing. **The post was already shared 200,000 times, and counting...**

For examples of the Facebook posts go to the full Report pages 6,7,8 reference below:

Ref: https://stopworldcontrol.com/downloads/en/vaccines/vaccinereport.pdf

Notice in the last comment how the lady says that everybody in the hospital is afraid to report this as a "vaccine" reaction, and another person says, 'the doctors can't report it'.

Note that not reporting adverse effects of these poisonous "vaccines" is a violation of the Hippocratic Oath. **All doctors not reporting adverse effects are liable to be struck off and perhaps face criminal prosecution.**

That is proof of what was explained earlier:

Most medical professionals are either too terrified to report adverse events, or they are simply corrupt. This causes the true prevalence of vaccine injuries to remain hidden from the world, which is powerful real-life evidence for what the **Lazarus report revealed: only 1% of vaccine injuries are reported to the authorities. The 250,000+ comments show that once people find a place to report suffering caused by the injections, we see a tsunami...**

It is Far Worse Than We Think

1. VAERS published 726,963 adverse events, including 15,386 deaths as of September 17, 2021
2. CDC fraud expert says that number of deaths is at least five times, and possibly ten times higher
3. A whistle-blower from the Centers for Medicare & Medicaid Service (CMS) revealed how almost 50,000 people died from the injections. They represent only 20% of the U.S. population, meaning that if this data is applied to the entire population 250,000 have died
4. 150,000 reports have been rejected or scrubbed by the VAERS system
5. The actual number of anaphylaxes is 50 to 120 times higher than claimed by the CDC

6. Everyone who dies before two weeks after the second injection, is not considered a vaccine death, which causes the majority of early vaccine deaths to be ignored
7. Moderna received over 300,000 reports of adverse events in only three months-time
8. The Lazarus Report shows that only 1% of adverse events is being reported by the public
9. The majority of the population is not aware of the existence of systems where they can report vaccine adverse events
10. Aggressive censorship and propaganda told the public that adverse events are rare, causing people to not understand how their health problems stem from past injections
11. The shaming and blaming of medical professionals who say anything against the "vaccines", cause many in the medical community to avoid reporting adverse events
12. The fear of being held accountable after administering an injection that killed or disabled patients, further prevents medical personnel from reporting it
13. Having accepted financial incentives to promote, and administer the "covid" "vaccines", also stops medical personnel from reporting adverse events
14. Profit driven vaccine manufacturers have every reason not to report the destruction their untested experimental products are causing
15. 250,000+ Facebook users comment about "vaccine" deaths and serious injuries

This alarming data leads world experts, like the Nobel Prize Winner in Medicine, Dr. Luc Montagnier, to issue a grave warning that we are currently facing the greatest risk of worldwide genocide, in the history of humanity.

Even the inventor of the mRNA technology, Dr. Robert Malone, warns against these injections that are using his technology [in a wrong way]. The situation is so severe that former Pfizer vice president and chief scientist Dr. Mike Yeadon came forward to warn humanity for these extremely dangerous injections. One of his best-known videos is titled 'A Final Warning'. Another world renown scientist, Geert Vanden Bossche, former Head of Vaccine Development Office in Germany, and Chief Scientific Officer at Univac, also risks his name and career, by bravely speaking out against administration of the "covid" shots. The vaccine developer warns that the injections can compromise the immunity of the vaccinated, making them vulnerable for every new variant. **World War II holocaust survivors wrote to the European Medicines Agency demanding the injections to be stopped, which they consider to be a new holocaust.**

In the European Union (which consists of only 27 of the 50 European countries) the official reports of EudraVigilance officially admit as of August 18th 2021, that approximately 22,000 people died and 2 million suffered side effects, of which 50% are serious. [Assuming linearity and extrapolating to the other 23 countries then we have 40,740 people died and 3.7 million suffered side effects, of which 50% i.e., 1.85M are serious throughout Europe's 50 countries.]

What are serious injuries?

'It be classified as 'serious' if it corresponds to a medical occurrence that results in death, is life threatening, requires inpatient hospitalisation, results in another medically important condition, or prolongation of existing hospitalisation, results in persistent or significant disability or incapacity, or is a congenital anomaly/birth defect.'

Adverse Effects in UK

Shortly before the national vaccination campaign started, the UK MHRA (Medicines and Healthcare Products Regulatory Agency) published the following request:

'The MHRA urgently seeks an Artificial Intelligence (AI) software tool to process the expected high volume of COVID-19 vaccine Adverse Drug Reaction (ADRs) and ensure that no details from the ADRs' reaction text are missed.'

The British government published a report of the first series of adverse events, including blindness, strokes, miscarriages, heart failure, paralysis, autoimmune disease, and more.

Shortly after the **first wave of immunization over 100,000 adverse events** were reported, including 1260 cases of loss of eyesight (including total blindness). The first part of the report praises the vaccines to be the best way to protect people from "COVID-19", and then continues to show the incredible destruction these vaccines are causing. **The hypocrisy is mindboggling.** Also, in the U.K. **miscarriages increased by 366% in only six weeks**, for "vaccinated" mothers.

Furthermore, the British Office for National Statistics inadvertently revealed that **30,305 people have died within 21 days of having the injection, during the first 6 months of 2021**. And a British scientist with 35 years of experience did an in-depth analysis of the **British Yellow Card reporting system and found it to be unreliable**.

'We can conclude that the Yellow Card reporting scheme can provide some limited information that may be useful for alerting the UK public to possible adverse effects of the "COVID-19" "vaccines". However, the initial conception of the scheme as a purely descriptive rather than as an experimental undertaking means that it cannot address the real issues that are of crucial importance to the UK public. These issues are whether there are causal relationships between "vaccination" with the PF [Pfizer] *and AZ* [AstraZeneca] *"vaccines" and serious adverse effects such as death, and if so, what are the size of these effects.'*

Strokes, Heart Attacks, Cancer...

A study by the University of San Francisco, or Salk Institute, shows that the "vaccines" turn the human body into a spike protein factory, making trillions of spikes that cause blood clots, which cause strokes and heart attacks. Another study confirms how the vaccines can cause deadly blood clots, that in turn cause heart attacks and strokes. The New England Journal of Medicine shows how the jabs cause heart inflammation, and the same journal published a study about the dramatic increase of [child] miscarriages. Several studies prove the reality of antibody dependent enhancement. **Also, the occurrence of infertility and reduced sperm count is confirmed. Lastly a study showed that the injections cause cancer.** And these are just a few examples...

Dr. Carrie Madej studied vaccines and transhumanism for two decades. In her documentary 'The Battle For Humanity', produced by Stop World Control, she warned that these [Covid19] **injections could permanently change the human DNA, with potentially disastrous outcomes**. Fact-checkers around the world - who are often paid by the "vaccine" industry - jumped to label it as fake news. Facebook made it their policy to censor all voices that warned how this gene therapy could potentially alter the human genome. Until... a Facebook employee recorded and released an insider zoom meeting with Facebook CEO Mark Zuckerberg, who told his staff that the injections do indeed change the human DNA!

These are Facebook CEO Mark Zuckerberg exact words:

'We just don't know the long-term side effects of basically modifying people's DNA and RNA to directly encode in a person's DNA and RNA, basically the ability to produce those antibodies and whether that causes other mutations or other risks downstream.'

Ref: Video: https://www.projectveritas.com/video/facebook-ceo-mark-zuckerberg-takes-anti-vax-stance-in-violation-of-his-own/

Ref: Article: https://thepostmillennial.com/project-veritas-leak-shows-mark-zuckerberg-violating-code/

The above Zuckerberg references provided by Daryl Brown of 'The No Corruption Alliance'

Ref: https://www.nocorruptionalliance.com/

Why do some people die, or become disabled for life, while others seem fine after being inoculated? Dr. Jane Ruby explains that not all vials have the same dosages. ClinicalTrials.gov shows that there are different phases of the "vaccination" experiment, with different dosages of the mRNA being administered to different people. An unknown percentage of the injections are even placebos!

This means that some people get a harmless substance injected, while others get a shot with 5, 10, 20, or 30 micrograms of mRNA.

Dr. Ruby warns that in the booster shots some vials contain as much as 100 or even 250 micrograms of mRNA. This explains why in certain areas the vaccinated seem fine, while in other areas **people drop dead after being injected. It's like Russian roulette: nobody knows what is being injected into their body! There is no informed consent.** If people however take the boosters, they will get different dosages. **Where previous shots may have been harmless, the next could be lethal.**

The excuse for murdering millions of people with these injections is that they supposedly prevent people from dying of "Covid". The reality is however that the so-called **number of "Covid" deaths is the greatest lie in history**. **Worldwide it was revealed that over 95% of all "Covid" deaths, were deaths from other causes.**

The Italian politician Vittorio Sgarbi exclaimed in the Italian Chamber of Deputies:

'Let's not make this the chamber of lies. Don't lie! Tell the truth. Don't say there's 25,000 dead. It's not true. Don't use the dead for rhetoric and terrorism. Figures from the Higher Institute of Health say 96.3% died of other diseases.' [other than "Covid19"]

Medical professionals around the world have testified of being pressured by their supervisors to report all patients as "Covid" and register every death - no matter what the cause was - as a "Covid" death. The internet has been flooded by thousands of testimonies of outraged people who said that they went to a doctor or hospital for issues unrelated to "COVID19" and to their amazement, they were registered as a "Covid" patient.

Dr. Elke de Klerk, founder of Doctors for Truth in the Netherlands, testified that she received secret messages in the dossiers of terminally ill patients, requesting that these people should be registered as "covid" deaths. Project Veritas called several funeral directors in New York, and they testified how every dead person was registered as "Covid", while everybody knew that was not correct. Minnesota senator Scott Jensen, who is also a practicing physician, revealed on Fox News that U.S. hospitals receive huge financial incentives to register patients as "Covid". **For every person they registered as a "Covid" death they are paid 39,000 US $Dollars**. This has been confirmed by medical professionals around the world. The technical director of CNN Charlie Chester was secretly filmed by a Project Veritas undercover journalist, while he admitted that **CNN inflated the death rates *'because fear sells'***.

New York was the epicentre of the "COVID-19" "pandemic".

In the heart of New York is the famous Elmhurst Hospital where patients who repeatedly tested negative for COVID-19 are still registered as 'confirmed COVID19'. They are put on a respirator in a "Covid" ward... which causes them to die. This was secretly filmed!

In a revealing documentary by Journeyman Pictures, this nurse talks about the crimes she constantly sees happening in Elmhurst Hospital. She shows on her smartphone how a patient indeed **tested negative for "COVID19" twice**... and yet was registered as 'confirmed' "COVID-19"'. **She explains that this happens all the time in Elmhurst Hospital: deception and murder resulting in high "COVID-19" mortality rates that are trumpeted by the media.**

Many more of these criminal horror stories could be included in this Chapter 11.

However, print space in this book does not permit it. For the full, illustrated and fully referenced report see the reference below:

Ref: https://stopworldcontrol.com/downloads/en/vaccines/vaccinereport.pdf

CHAPTER 12

CONFIDENCE TRICK 12: MAINSTREAM MEDIA REPORTED NEWS – THEY DID NOT - THEY ARE PUPPETS OF PSEUDO "PANDEMIC" PSYCHOLOGICAL PROPAGANDA

Proof That The
"Pandemic" Was Planned
With A Purpose

Lawyers & Experts Reveal Evidence for World Dictatorship Under the Guise of "Pandemics"

Among the expert witnesses are World Health Organization advisors, a United Nations official, members of British Intelligence Services, former officers from the U.S. and U.K. military, an expert from the USA Centre for Disease Control, a former vice-president from Pfizer, a Nobel prize winner for medicine, and many other high-level witnesses

Some of the Organisations represented:

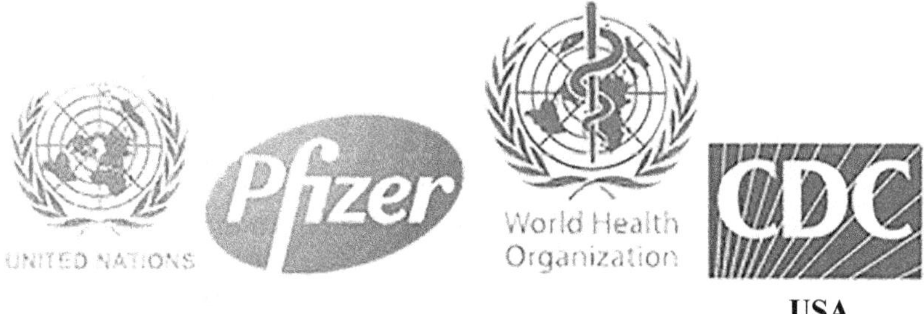

USA

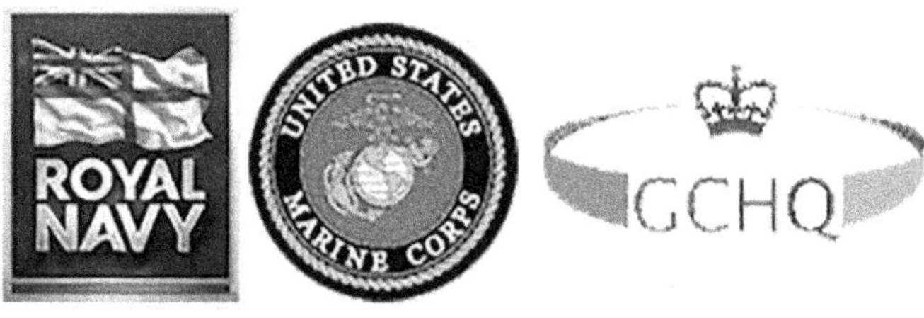

UK **UK**

Ref: **https://stopworldcontrol.com/proof/**

The World Health Organization WHO has a plan for ten years of infectious diseases says a WHO virologist

Documents that announced the coronavirus pandemic:

Scenarios for the Future by The Rockefeller Foundation
A futuristic Scenario by John Hopkins Centre [USA]
Australian Health Management Plan for Pandemic Influenza
WHO Instructed the World to Prepare for Imminent Coronavirus Pandemic
Global "Pandemic" Methodologies

Psychological Manipulation

The experts show how mind control, psychological manipulation and hypnosis techniques are used to control the opinions and behaviour of the public worldwide. The information is backed up with official documents issued by the governments and the named organizations. Below is one example of an **official document from the British Government**, revealing an official strategy to psychologically manipulate the public – **taken from UK Government SAGE / SPI_B "Covid" Team Minutes**:

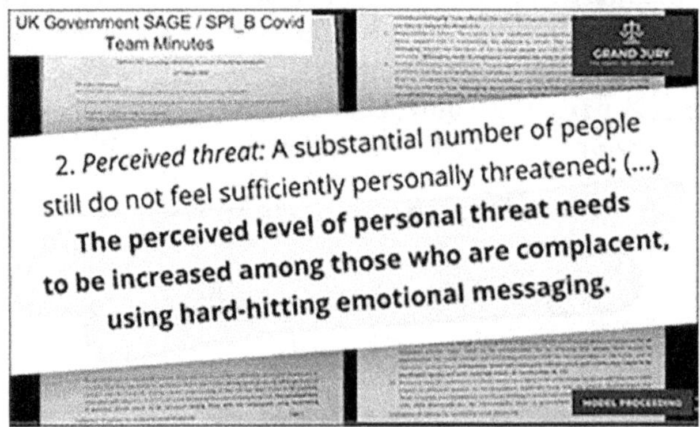

Global Lockstep Media Propaganda

The history of the Global Media from December 2019 until 2022 is clear. Any voice that was not in tune with the mainstream narrative was silenced or side-lined. Many leading scientists and medical staff were banned from the mainstream media and social media platforms if they dared to offer an alternative view despite it being backed up by scientific evidence. Dr Robert Malone (mRNA architect), Dr Vernon Coleman, Dr Sam White (also lost his license to practice – reinstated under Common Law) Robert F. Kennedy Jr (Trial Lawyer/Big Pharma Prosecutor and nephew of ex-President John F Kennedy) and many, many others the world over were banned from all social media platforms. **Never before in World History has the world's main organs of media been so homogeneous and synchronised in the pursuit of a common lie**. The Holy Grail was a mantra of "virus" "SarsCov2" "Covid19" "pandemic" "lockdown" "social distancing" "masks" "PCR Tests" "vaccinations" – people in UK were even "educated" about how they should wash their hands. All of this was blasted across the world unsupported by even one scientific study worthy of the name being a tenth the way to its completion! It was clear that this was being conceived and organised at a trans-global level above the jurisdictions of democratically elected sovereign states.

The mainstream media in UK and worldwide was merely a pawn in the Game, as were the so called "world leaders".

USA Judge Orders Fauci to Cough It Up

Ref: https://brownstone.org/articles/judge-orders-fauci-to-cough-it-up/?utm_medium=one signal&utm_source=push

A lawsuit against the federal government – Dr Anthony Fauci in particular – from the Attorneys General of Missouri and Louisiana has been brewing for a good part of the summer of 2022. The issue concerns the **censoring of certain high-level experts on social media**, three of whom are senior scholars of the Brownstone Institute. We know for sure that this censorship began early in the pandemic response and included exchanges between Fauci and then head of USA NIH Francis Collins, who called for a **"quick and devastating takedown"** of the '**Great Barrington Declaration**'.

Great Barrington Declaration

Mission Statement

'As infectious disease epidemiologists and public health scientists we have grave concerns about the damaging physical and mental health impacts of the prevailing "COVID-19" policies and recommend an approach we call Focused Protection.'

Ref: https://gbdeclaration.org/

At issue for the USA Judge is whether and to what extent the government itself has had a hand in encouraging tech companies [social media companies: Google, Facebook, Twitter etc] to **squelch speech rights**. **If so, this is unconstitutional. It flies in the face of the First Amendment** [USA]. It never should have happened. That it did require arduous legal means to expose and, hopefully, stop.

The First Amendment framers guaranteed that Congress would make no law **"abridging the freedom of speech, or of the press."** The Constitution never allowed an exception for an administrative bureaucracy answerable not even to voters, to collaborate with large-scale private corporations, to obtain the same exception result by other means. This has been, and still is worldwide, **an extraordinary violation of free speech**.

'Doctors for Information'

A group of almost **one thousand medical doctors** in Germany called 'Doctors for Information', which is supported by more than **7,000 professionals** including attorneys, scientists, teachers etc., made a shocking statement during a national press conference:

'The Corona panic is a play. It's a scam. A swindle. It's high time we understood that we're in the midst of a global crime.'

This large group of medical experts publishes a newspaper with circulation of **500,000 copies every week,** to alert the public about the **misinformation in the mainstream media** about the **"coronavirus"**. They also organize mass protests with millions of people throughout Europe.

Ref: https://expose-news.com/?s=doctors+for+information

'Doctors for Truth'

In Spain, a group of **600 medical doctors** called **'Doctors for Truth'** made a similar statement during a press conference:

Ref: https://medicalkidnap.com/2020/10/18/doctors-for-truth-tens-of-thousands-medical-professionals-suing-and-calling-for-end-to-covid-tyranny/

'"Covid-19" is a false pandemic created for political purposes. This is a world dictatorship with a sanitary excuse. We urge doctors, the media and political authorities to stop this criminal operation by spreading the truth.'

'World Doctors Alliance'

'Doctors for Information' and 'Doctors for Truth' have joined forces with similar groups of practitioners around the world in the **'World Doctors Alliance'**

Ref: https://worlddoctorsalliance.com/

This historic alliance connects more than one hundred thousand medical professionals around the world. **They reveal how the "pandemic" is the greatest crime in history and offer solid scientific evidence for this claim.** ***They also take legal actions against governments who are playing along with this criminal operation.***

Ref: https://stopworldcontrol.com/proof/

'World Freedom Alliance'

Similarly, the World Freedom Alliance was formed - a network of attorneys, medical experts, politicians, bankers, and many other professionals who are working together to **expose the 'Covid Crime'**, and who are starting to build a new world of freedom. ***They want to make sure these kinds of worldwide scams that destroy millions of lives can never occur again.***

Ref: **https://worldfreedomalliance.org/**

Lawyers & Experts Reveal Evidence for World Dictatorship Under the Guise of "Pandemics"

The evidence is presented during six Grand Jury legal proceedings, that each last about six hours. The length of these proceedings, make it hard for the majority of the public to receive this information. That's why ***Stop World Control*** is creating easy-to-read summaries of each six-hour session, so these extremely important revelations can reach a greater audience. The first summary is now available and can be downloaded for free.

Ref: https://stopworldcontrol.com/jury/

'The No Corruption Alliance'

Quote:

'The No Corruption Alliance wants [UK] parliament and our executive government branch to be governed by a majority of independents who demonstrate that they are committed to serving the interests of their people instead of their political party and their big donors.

We think we can achieve this, at least in part, by unifying ourselves under the banner of preventing corruption. We provide a directory of independent candidates who have signed a pledge designed to prevent corruption and demonstrate that they are serious about putting their people first, and we also list local branches that they may be connected to. This directory also provides easily accessible tools to help you vet those candidates.

We hold no views or judgements on candidates' policies or morals. Our aim is simply to provide an easy to navigate directory and tackle corruption to ensure that our democracy is healthier, stronger, and engaged. We hope to help in bridging some of the gaps that make it challenging to get independents elected to parliament up to this point. We want to change that.

The directory also provides the ability to help you connect with others in your region too, with the options to message others as well as listing information of regular meetups in person.

We provide many resources and sources of useful information as well as run a blog. The blog aims to commit a laser-focus on pinpointable areas of embedded systematic corruption and provide an attached suggestable solution within each article's conclusion. We aim to abide by this laser focus on accurately described baked-in corruption facts and not descend into personal attack-based propaganda for the sake of such. Equally we hope that this solution-focused approach extends to our community and beyond. We hope that the blog will be transferable into a physical magazine at some point in the not-too-distant future.

This community could also be used as a massive force to ensure that our general election system remains fair. This vigilance could also be extended to our other election systems too.

It is amazing what can be overcome if all the different peoples of our land are able to unite alongside our common goals to defeat the festering corruption that is kneecapping our beautiful humankind.'

Unquote.

[Note: **'The No Corruption Alliance'** model is applicable to any country in the world where the people want to be represented by honourable, true, honest men and women of indubitable integrity and faith in the possibilities for a better world future for the many, not for a world as currently enforced, which is for the few at the expense of the many.]

Ref: https://www.nocorruptionalliance.com/

Also, Ref: Appendix I – PDF Download File page 47 as per below:

The whole of the UK Covid19 policy and the "vaccination" policy has been carried out by the **British Cabinet Office**. ***"over 1.5M adverse effects from vaccines...vaccines deaths outstrip the dangers of "Covid19"...We have a team of gangsters in power...misuse applied psychology practices...to mislead the public and change their behaviour..."***

Ref: https://odysee.com/@GrandJury:f/Grand-Jury-Day-2-online_1:f hrs:mins:secs 2:16:0 – 2:20:01

Dr. Reiner Fuellmich is the Founder and Chairman of the 'Corona Investigative Committee' also Founder 'International Crime Investigative Committee' 'ICIC' and a world-renowned trial lawyer with almost three decades of experience in successfully suing large fraudulent corporations, like Deutsche Bank, Volkswagen, etc.

During the "COVID-19" "pandemic" Dr. Fuellmich observed criminal practices committed by media and governments worldwide. He founded the 'Corona Investigative Committee' and began an extensive investigation, during which he interviewed over 150 experts from all fields of science. Many of these experts are recognized as world leaders in their field of expertise. Together with other lawyers from around the world, Dr. Fuellmich gathered undeniable evidence that this **"Covid19" "pandemic" is a series of unprecedented crimes against humanity**.

Dr. Fuellmich, ten international lawyers, and a judge decided to present the evidence for these crimes against humanity to the public during a grand jury proceeding. Among the eyewitnesses are former members of the British Intelligence Services, the UK Royal Navy, the US Marine Corps, the World Health Organization, the United Nations, a former vice-president from Pfizer, a Nobel Prize winner for medicine, and many more high-level experts.

What is a Grand Jury

In serious criminal cases in the U.S. a grand jury is presented with the evidence at hand to convince them that this evidence is sufficient to bring public charges against the defendants. **We, the people of the world, are adopting this model to prove to the public, with the help of witnesses, lawyers, a judge, and experts from around the world, that we are dealing with crimes against humanity that span the globe.**

The allegation is that the world's governments have come under the controlling influence of globalist corrupt and criminal power structures. The power structures colluded to stage a global "pandemic" that they had been planning for years.

To this end, they deliberately created mass panic through false statements of fact and a socially engineered psychological operation whose messages they conveyed through the corporate media. The purpose of this mass panic was to persuade the population to agree to **experimental so-called "vaccinations" - which they are not. These have been proven to be neither effective nor safe, but extremely dangerous and even lethal.**

The investigation serves as a model proceeding to secure indictments against some of the criminally and civilly responsible figureheads of these crimes against humanity.

A secondary purpose is to create awareness about the factual collapse of the current hijacked system and its institutions, and, as a consequence, awareness of:

- the necessity of the people themselves retaking their sovereignty,
- the necessity of first stopping the measures by refusing to comply,
- and the necessity of jump-starting the people's own new systems of health care, education, economics, and judiciary, so that democracy and the rule of law on the basis of our Constitutions will be re-established.

[Currently there are six names of the persons/organisations that have been announced for prosecution – August 2022:

Bill Gates Bill and Melinda Gates Foundation
Dr Fauci Chief Medical Advisor to President USA, Director of NIAID
Tedros Adhanom Ghebreyesus Director-General of the World Health Organization WHO
Dr Drosten Researcher/Designer [worthless] PCR Tests – Chapter 8
Pfizer Pharmaceutical Corporation
Blackrock Investment Management Company]

Transcript Summary

The purpose of this **Grand Jury Summary** is to make the most important information revealed by the expert witnesses accessible to as many people as possible. We have focused on those facts that reveal what is really going on in our world, to help the public understand the graveness of the current world crisis. Those who want to get the full spectrum of details, please watch the full video sessions here:

Ref: https://stopworldcontrol.com/downloads/GrandJurySummary1.pdf

This document is part one of five Grand Jury Summaries. It contains critical information from Day 2, titled **'The General Historic and Geopolitical Backdrop to All of This'**. This may well be the most important session of the entire Grand Jury proceeding, as it exposes how a masterplan has been created to achieve total world domination under the guise of health emergencies. The Opening Statements are not included, as they are too lengthy and can easily be viewed on the website:

Ref: https://stopworldcontrol.com/jury/

Defending Humanity

We encourage every reader to distribute this **Grand Jury Summary** within their community. The criminal power structures rely entirely on the ignorance of the people. Once the public becomes informed, they shift from unquestioning compliance to intelligent resistance. Therefore, the single most important action we can all take is to inform others. We must especially educate all those who have a position of influence in our communities. Send this **Grand Jury Summary**, either in digital or printed form, to school directors and teachers, hospital directors and medical staff, law enforcement officers, lawyers and judges, pastors, mayors and commissioners, local media editors and journalists.

This information really needs to reach all those in a position of public service. These members of our societies are unknowingly the minions of the criminals, as they blindly follow orders that directly lead to the death of millions of people, and the permanent damaging of hundreds of millions of lives. Once all our public servants people understand what is really going on, they will stop being the extensions of the criminal hands, lest they become consciously complicit.

If we don't stand up and act now, we may forever lose the ability to do so, as the World Economic Forum WEF is preparing to install global governance over the flow of information and the internet and will attempt to forever shut the mouth of all who value the freedom of humanity. If there ever was a time for all to rise and act, it is now.

The editor,
David J. Sörensen
https://stopworldcontrol.com/

The City of London Summary

The expert witnesses during session 2 of the Grand Jury are a former officer of the British Intelligence Services (partner agency to the US National Security Agency), and a Canadian investigative journalist. They explain the long history of the aim for world dominance by the British elite. The British Empire still exists, and includes the United Kingdom, Canada, Australia, New Zealand, India, 19 African Countries, and the Caribbean, while they extend their hand into virtually every other nation of the world. Their headquarters are in the City of London, an area of one square mile, which is the financial centre of the world. The City of London Corporation isn't governed by the British government but on the contrary reigns supreme over it. The City of London Corporation has its own courts and police and has never been challenged in its sovereignty and self-government. It rules over the Crown and over most of the Earth.

The British elite, [part of the Evil300] believe they have the right to enslave the rest of humanity, which they consider to be their 'livestock' or 'cattle' [perhaps also 'useless eaters']. In their views they own the population - body, mind and soul. Democracy is only an illusion to keep the people at peace, while the City of London calls the shots and pulls the strings.

This "elite" made several attempts at so-called 'New World Orders', which all failed. They almost succeeded in reigning in the United States but failed there as well. Now they use the "COVID-19" "pandemic" to further their goal of world domination, using psychological techniques to get the world population to blindly obey their every command, under the guise of 'keeping everybody safe'.

Mind control has for a long time been at the heart of their strategy. After three industrial revolutions, a fourth industrial revolution is now emerging that focuses on owning the minds of the people.

The deeper purpose of the **"vaccination" programs is to edit the genome of humanity**, [and gain total global control and de-populate the planet] and thus create a new trans-human race that will behave according to the desires of the oligarchs. This has always been the ultimate desire of tyrants in the past, but only now does technology allow the re-creation of humanity to become the perfect slaves.

Our world is threatened by a rebirth of the ancient system of slavery, which has been technologically upgraded to install a whole new level of all-encompassing slavery over the entire world population.

The City of London is the financial heart of the British Empire and the dominant power in the world. It readied itself for that situation from roughly 1870. The modern world, the monopolization, the cartelization of the world, begins at that time. Everything that we do in investigating the corruption emanating from British Crown monopolies and City of London money does seem to point back to this period from around 1870, in which there were several revolutions by the British elite.

There was a revolution in what you might call mind space, which since 2010 has been an explicit term used by the British government's central department, the Cabinet Office.

- A revolution in the quality of education offered to British and other Western schoolchildren.
- A revolution in the theft of intellectual property by the elite.
- A revolution in the model of healthcare and free access to it.
- At home, a constitutional revolution from the classic British Liberal democracy model.

This all happened since 1870, and in Britain it was largely complete by the crucial year 1947-1948 when Britain had a unique situation of a National Health Service and was pushing the way towards the military unification of the European continent and the whole of North Atlantic Treaty Organisation 'NATO'.

The Cabinet Office is a department which was set up in the early 20th century, as the repository of Crown prerogatives. From around 1870, the constitutional revolution has ensured that financiers controlling political parties actually pull the levers of Crown prerogatives. Behind the scenes, the model of government Britain still is that of an inner sanctum, the Privy Council, which actually governs in the name of The Crown.

The history academic at Georgetown University, Carroll Quigley, former tutor of Bill Clinton, wrote in his book, *'Tragedy & Hope: A History of the World in Our Time'*, that there have been four industrial revolutions. Yes, that familiar language coming from the World Economic Forum WEF was being written about in the 1960s already by Quigley. The perspective which is being assumed here is that of who owns the population, first in Britain and then in the British Empire.

- First revolution: the ownership of land, of agricultural means provides wealth
- Second revolution: mechanical - industrial
- Third revolution: in which financial capital dominates the world.

It's from this period around 1870 onwards that the smart money in the City of London realizes that even that bubble is going to burst.

Just one example of the total reach of British intelligence in areas which is not constitutionally able or permitted to have, is that MI5, even before the Second World War, was vetting who got onto the airwaves of the BBC, who got promoted and who got transferred. It was set up by the nobility bloodlines to further their private aims.

The British Cabinet Office is openly speaking about its control of the world's thinking and the thinking of the British people. They're labelling parts of the brain under the label of MINDSPACE. The cover of the Mindpsace document is shown below:

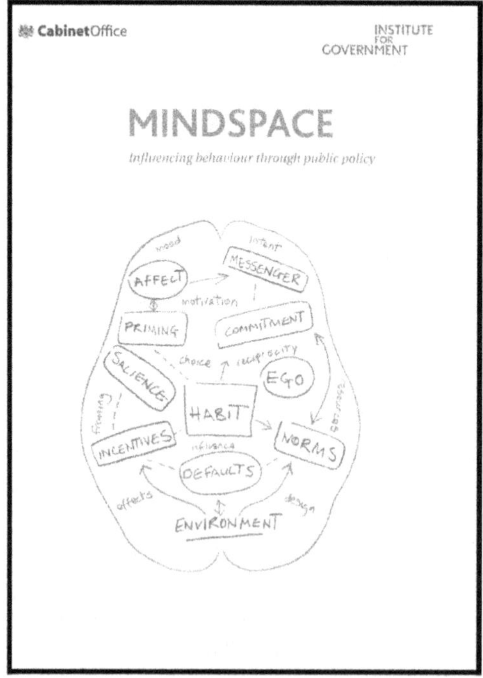

Ref: https://www.instituteforgovernment.org.uk/publications/mindspace

Their document says: *'Even if people agree with the behaviour goal, they may object to the means of accomplishing it. The different MINDSPACE effects will attract different levels of controversy. There are several factors that determine controversy.'*

Owning The People

'The goal is therefore to make sure that citizens don't fully realize that their behaviour is being changed, or at least how it is being changed.'

Below is a transcript of the Chairman, Reiner Fuellmich, Grand Jury discussions with Alex Thomson, Dexter L-J. Ryneveldt Attorney and N. Ana Garner Attorney at Law, USA

Grand Jury Proceeding by the Peoples' Court of Public Opinion

Reiner Fuellmich - Chairman: *'Another thing that I wanted to clarify is, you mentioned that it is just a few families who really run the City of London. You mentioned the names of Rothschild and Rhodes and Astor. Is it true that it's just a few families who are trying to dominate the world through the City of London?'*

Alex Thomson - Expert Witness, former Officer of Britain's Signal Intelligence Agency: *'Yes. I have never found better material than that of a writing duo which is Dutch/German American. The Dutchman is Robin de Ruiter. His American German co-author is Fritz Springmeier from South Carolina. They have the rather shocking book titled* ***'Bloodlines of the Illuminati'****. But their work is solid.'*

'They consistently show that the City of London, Manhattan, the European continent, are very much dominated by a small number of families.'

Alex Thomson: *'Often 13 is given as the top level of these families. Obviously, there are levels below that. The French, for example, often spoke about "les 200 families," the 200 bloodlines, that run the deep state. But the senior ones terrorize the junior ones...'*

Reiner Fuellmich: *'Did I hear correctly that you used the term livestock? Is that really the view that these people have of the rest of the world?'*

Alex Thomson: *'It is explicitly the view that, certainly in the 1990s when I was at a senior British boarding school, this term was used by the grandsons of City of London seniors. They used the word 'livestock' to describe the British population.'*

[They [the people] are considered 'cattle'/'livestock'/'useless eaters' and do not deserve a place in the world other than under the direction of the global "elite"/Evil300.]

Dexter L-J. Ryneveldt Attorney: *'So, you will agree that financial dominance is at the core of the "Covid-19" "pandemic"?'*

Alex Thomson: *'Yes, I would, and I would qualify it very slightly by reminding you that in Carroll Quigley's summary of the Anglo-American elite establishment's worldview, he points out that the ownership of financial assets is already outdated by the 1960s. And he knows that the great brains, not necessarily the good brains, a century prior to him already saw this coming.'*

They regard the real wealth as human minds and health and the ability to alter and copyright, in time, the human being into a new model that would behave as required and expected.

N. Ana Garner Attorney at Law, USA: '*You mention copyrighting the human mind, copyrighting even the genetics. Do you feel that there is a link between the current so-called "vaccines" – the shots from Pfizer, Moderna, Janssen, AstraZeneca – and this goal of copyrighting the humans?'*

Alex Thomson: *'I very strongly believe that. I'm not medically or biotechnologically qualified to explain how much truth there may be in this, but I've seen time and again that where there is hype and where there is a pseudo theological belief among the "elite" in Britain and America that you can achieve a certain aim by pulling a certain trick - such as by editing a gene and stamping a copyright on the human body - that is enough motivation in and of itself to fuel a serious attempt to go that way.'*

Ref: https://odysee.com/@WrongthinkInc:e/Grand-Jury-Day-2-Englishrehosted:4 hrs: mins:secs 00:01:02-00:46:53:

CHAPTER 13

CONFIDENCE TRICK 13: UK CORONAVIRUS ACT 2020 WAS LAWFUL – UNLIKELY

'It appears that our Governments do not have a problem with experimenting on our elderly, on our Police Officers, on our First Response Staff, on our Doctors and Nurses, on our General Public and now apparently don't have problem experimenting on our children'

Dr Richard Fleming PhD, MD, JD
Distinguished Physician & Doctor of Law USA
6th August 2022

Ref: https://australiaoneparty.com/truth-about-covid-coming-out-now/

The quote above is given at timing c. 48:24 mins:secs in the interview URL above.

Despotic laws can — even should — be ignored, says Jonathan Sumption Justice of the UK Supreme Court Rtd

The retired Justice of the Supreme Court admits breaking lockdown regulations

In an interview Jonathan Sumption retired Justice of The Supreme Court admitted breaking the lockdown regulations. 'I don't accept that there is a moral obligation to comply with the law,'

[Is there anyone who has read a line of Ethics worth reading (i.e., Immanuel Kant) and studied the "Covid" business with a open mind, who would disagree?]

Further Lord Sumption stated:

'Sometimes the most public-spirited thing that you can do with despotic laws like these* [“Covid19” Mandates] *is to ignore them.'

Ref: https://www.spectator.co.uk/article/despotic-laws-can-even-should-be-ignored-says-jonathan-sumption

The author contends that:

The UK Coronavirus Act 2020 is open to challenge in its basic premise, in its fundamental principles and in its actualities regarding the lawfulness of actions undertaken under its umbrella

<u>There was never a "pandemic"</u>.

It is clear that "Covid19" has much the same fatality rate (c. 0.14% of population) as the Common Flu which we have annually. This clearly demonstrates that the UK "Covid19" Mandates, implemented under the UK Coronavirus Act 2020 were not reasonable, proportionate, appropriate, nor necessary.

As stated previously in Chapter 1:

Sars-Cov-2 DOES NOT and NEVER HAS, ACTUALLY EVER EXISTED!! The so called "virus" was NOT a Sars virus!! <u>Indeed, the so called "virus" WAS NOT A VIRUS AT ALL!!</u>

Results of Studies by Dr Poornima Wagh PhD Santa Barbara CA, USA confirm this!

Dr Poornima Wagh, Researcher, 2 PhDs in Virology and Immunology, Santa Barbara, CA, USA

Quote:

***"How do you find HIV spike proteins in a 'NOVEL' virus genome? You don't, it's called <u>FRAUD</u>"* [What has been called, by WHO etc. "Sars-Cov-2" <u>IS NOT</u> a virus!]**

"Studies of true isolation* [Koch Postulates] *from April to September 2020 using tests repeated three times with 1,500 samples resulted in only debris being found! NO "Sars-Cov2/Covid19" or any other virus was found" "Studies repeated in 7 Universities – same results"

The samples failed the Koch Postulates Examination. Viruses exist in nature, if no virus was found, then the so-called "virus" does not exist in nature and therefore it must be <u>something man-made</u>. If man-made then it is a <u>Bioweapon</u>* [perhaps <u>Chemical weapon</u>] *(because of the use of GAIN of FUNCTION (see Dr Robert Malone below) and the harm it has caused by lockdowns, masks, social distancing in physical and economic terms – See Report) and its deliberate use between 2019-2022 is indicative of <u>mass murder and Genocide</u>.

Dr Robert Malone, The architect of mRNA and RNA as a drug discusses the INTERNATIONAL COVID SUMMIT and other items:

He states: *'In USA FDA AND CDC are acting beyond the law, 'Covid-19' originated in a laboratory using GAIN of FUNCTION technology, "vaccinated" are at the highest risk from covid spreading, in Israel "vaccinated" are getting infected-they then go to hospital and DIE, the SOCIAL CONTRACT will be destroyed.'*

Ref: https://www.youtube.com/watch?v=EWWvk2SaMS4

[Israel at the early stages of the "pandemic" was the most vaccinated and fastest vaccinated country in the world per capita yet had the most post "vaccinated" "covid" infections!! "Covid" infections rising from cumulative total of 131,317 on 6th September 2020 to 4.64M on 5th September 2022 an increase of 35 times over two years!!]

Ref: https://ourworldindata.org/coronavirus/country/israel

There was a very interesting legal case in Alberta, Canada that sets a precedent under UK law. A man was prosecuted under the Canadian equivalent of UK Coronavirus Act 2020 (Alberta Public Health Act), he was fined $1,200 under that law because he was in a public place with a group of more than10 people. He challenged the prosecution and because the prosecution lawyers could not produce evidence to the court that ***"Sars-Cov2/Covid19"*** **HAD been isolated**, it is claimed that the case was dismissed and the "Covid19" mandates in Alberta, Canada were overturned and immediately stopped. No more lockdowns, "vaccinations", masks, social distancing, contact tracing etc. ALL "Covid19" MANDATES STOPPED, it is claimed.

On 4th May 2021 the defendant Mr Patrick King requested evidence from Deena Hinshaw, Chief Medical Officer of Health to be produced in court that ***"Sars-Cov2"*** had been isolated. Claims to isolation of "Sars-Cov2" are NOT valid unless samples are taken from patients proven to have "SarsCov2/Covid19" and the "virus" is isolated [by centrifugal techniques] and then subjected to the test using Koch postulates. Mr King was clear in his request as detailed verbatim from the court document below:

'I request all white papers describing the isolation of the COVID-19 aka SARS-CoV-2 virus in human beings, directly from a sample taken from a diseased patient, where the patient sample was not first combined with any other source of genetic material. Note: The word "isolate" indicates: a thing is separated from all other material surrounding I am not requesting white papers where "isolation" of SARS-CoV-2 refers to: - the culturing of something, or - the performance of an amplification test (PCR), or - the sequencing of something. To clarify I am requesting via disclosure all white papers showing Isolation of the SARS-CoV-2 virus in human beings in your possession or in the possession of Alberta Health Ministry, as these white papers would have been integral in the crafting of the statutes made under the "Public Health Act" here in Alberta.'

Since Mr King was self-representing the Judge was obliged to advocate for him and duly advise him on court procedures. The judge allowed Mr King to subpoena Deena Hinshaw, Chief Medical Officer for Health, Alberta. Three days after the subpoena an officer visited Mr King and asked for his address, email, and phone number – information he already had many times on court documents! Finally, the officer said: ***"I am here to tell you that your court case has been cancelled."*** Later Mr King was subpoenaed by Deena Hinshaw's lawyers on a Sunday morning at 11.53 to appear in court in less than 24 hours which is a court procedural violation!

Mr King: ***'I knew that they were up to something.'***

The court agreed that this was a procedural violation on the part of Deena Hinshaw, Chief Medical Officer of Health's lawyers. **Since when does a Government official's lawyers invoke a Court procedural violation?** Mr King offered to hold the court session on the Wednesday 24th July, but the judge retorted No we can't because Deena Hinshaw's lawyers cannot supply the information you request. The court case then, in effect, went from Deena Hinshaw v Mr Patrick King **to the Office of Her Majesty the Queen (Queen Elizabeth II, (Buckingham Palace, London SW1A 1AA UK)) v Mr Patrick King. In this case 'The Crown' was requested to provide material evidence to the Court that the SARS-CoV-2 "virus" had been isolated (as described above). The UK Crown could not provide the evidence required to the Court! All Covid19 mandates, lockdowns, vaccines, masks, isolations etc. etc. were dropped it is claimed.** See Appendix V

Ref: https://www.redvoicemedia.com/2021/08/freedom-fighter-court-victory-ends-masking-shots-quarantine-in-alberta/?utm_sou [page not found happened recently – we know not why]

In this Court case, with Canada being part of the British Commonwealth, and the head of the Commonwealth, The Crown could not provide the Court in Alberta, Canada with the required material evidence, implies that the UK Coronavirus Act 2020 is also open to challenge as to its lawfulness if the UK Government and its authorities SAGE, GMC, NHS, MHRA and every Intellect in The Commonwealth etc. cannot provide such material evidence reports confirming that the SARS-CoV-2 "virus" has been isolated.

It has been reported that as for the isolation of the virus, in Canada, researchers at the Sunnybrook Research Institute, McMaster University and the University of Toronto reported in an article published in 2020 that "SarsCov2" had been isolated.

CORONA ACCOUNTABILITY (Covid19) 2022 organisation contacted these institutions by email for confirmation that they had truly isolated "Sars-Cov2":

'Your Institution has made claims that some of your researcher(s) has/have isolated "Sars-Cov2".

Please confirm that your procedures used Koch postulates, using purified samples from infected patients with true and correct symptoms.

Thank you.

Please reply within 2 days.

CORONA ACCOUNTABILITY (Covid19) 2022
18th August 2022'

No replies have been received!

The research paper makes NO reference to using Koch postulates. It is well known throughout the world of research in the field of virology that Koch postulates methodology is the gold standard test for testing for proof of the existence of a "virus" once the preliminary work of separating the "virus" from all other matter in the samples has been accomplished.

At the foot of the paper it states: *'Articles from Emerging Infectious Diseases are provided here courtesy of Centers for Disease Control and Prevention* [CDC] '

Research paper Ref: https://www.ncbi.nlm.nih.gov/pmc/articles/PMC7454076/

We have seen the attitude towards the truth of Robert Redfield CDC as described by Dr Wagh in Chapter 1:

Dr Wagh asked Robert Redfield, CDC Director, USA if he could assist her team's studies by providing samples. Robert Redfield could not provide samples to Dr Poornima Wagh and her researchers for testing in the laboratories and told the researchers to **call whatever they found "Sars-Cov-2"!!** Robert Redfield in giving this instruction was clearly acting, if not unlawfully, then certainly not within professional and ethical guidelines.

Furthermore, the persons listed below were requested for proof of the isolation of "Sars-Cov2" on three separate occasions in June, August and October 2022 **but with only two replies, NONE were in the affirmative.**

<u>Recipient</u>	**Office** (at the time – 2019/2020 onwards)
Boris Johnson	**Prime Minister**
Matt Hancock	**Health & Social Care**
Nadhim Zahawi	**"Covid" "Vaccine" Deployment**
Michael Gove	**Cabinet Office**
Sajid Javid	**Health & Social Care**
Suella Braverman	**Attorney General**
Priti Patel	**Home Office**
Baroness Hallett	**Chair Covid Inquiry 2021-**
Christopher Whitty	**Chief Medical Officer/Chief Medical Advisor**
Patrick Vallance	**Chief Scientific Advisor**
June Munro Raine	**CEO MHRA** - Medicines and Healthcare Products Regulatory Agency
Charlie Massey	**CEO GMC** – General Medical Council
Amanda Pritchard	**CEO NHS** – National Health Service
Neil Ferguson	**Researcher** - Imperial College, London

Furthermore, as stated above, it has been reported that circa 203 requests all over the world for scientific study results for "Sars-Cov-2" **isolation/purification** has resulted in **<u>zero claims</u>** of such isolation/purification. The countries totalled over 30 and included: Australia, Canada, New Zealand, UK, USA, South Africa, Norway, Portugal, Italy, India, etc. **<u>All reported *"No Record Found"*</u> [of true "Sars-Cov-2" isolation/purification.]**

It cannot be lawful, in any country that has any pretence to respect for law and order, for an enormous program of "vaccines" and "vaccination" of entire populations including children can be implemented and based on "laws" and "mandates" where the offending "virus" has not even been truly identified as existent by proper scientific isolation!! **This is not law and order; it is "healthcare" Fascism/Totalitarianism, which has nothing to do with healthcare.**

Laws must be reasonable, proportionate, necessary, appropriate otherwise it is bad law!!

The authorities must refute and rebut the allegations in this book in order for UK Coronavirus Act 2020 to be lawful!!

Below are the first few statements of the UK Coronavirus Act 2020 quoted verbatim:

Coronavirus Act 2020
2020 CHAPTER 7

An Act to make provision in connection with coronavirus; and for connected purposes **X1**

[25th March 2020]

Be it enacted by the Queen's most Excellent Majesty, [now King's most Excellent Majesty] by and with the advice and consent of the Lords Spiritual and Temporal, and Commons, in this present Parliament assembled, and by the authority of the same, as follows: —

PART 1
Main provisions

Interpretation

1. Meaning of "coronavirus" and related terminology

(1) In this Act—
- "coronavirus" means severe acute respiratory syndrome coronavirus 2 (SARS-CoV2);
- "coronavirus disease" means COVID-19 (the official designation of the disease which can be caused by coronavirus).

(2) A reference in this Act to infection or contamination, however expressed, is a reference to infection or contamination with coronavirus.

(3) But a reference in this Act to persons infected by coronavirus, however expressed, does not (unless a contrary intention appears) include persons who have been infected but are clear of coronavirus (unless re-infected).

As stated on previous pages:

Sars-Cov-2 DOES NOT and NEVER HAS, ACTUALLY EVER EXISTED!! The so called "virus" was NOT a Sars virus!! Indeed, the so called "virus" WAS NOT A VIRUS AT ALL!!

Results of Studies by Dr Poornima Wagh PhD Santa Barbara CA, USA confirm this!

Dr Poornima Wagh, Researcher, 2 PhDs in Virology and Immunology, Santa Barbara, CA, USA

Quote:

'How do you find HIV spike proteins in a 'NOVEL' virus genome? You don't, it's called FRAUD" **[What has been called, by WHO etc. "Sars-Cov-2" IS NOT a virus!]**

'Studies of true isolation **[Koch Postulates]** ***from April to September 2020 using tests repeated three times with 1,500 samples resulted in only debris being found! NO "Sars-Cov2/Covid19" or any other virus was found' 'Studies repeated in 7 Universities – same results'***

Dr Wagh *"there is no Sars-Cov2"*

Ref: https://www.bitchute.com/video/btuJXs0glmla/

If the research by Dr Poornima Wagh, Researcher, 2 PhDs in Virology and Immunology, Santa Barbara, CA, USA is correct, then perhaps there is a problem with the lawfulness of the UK Coronavirus Act 2020 as shown above.

Can the persons responsible for the UK Coronavirus Act 2020 refute the research by Dr Poornima Wagh and her results and unequivocally confirm that "coronavirus" which means severe acute respiratory syndrome coronavirus 2 (SARS-CoV2) as stated in the Coronavirus Act 2020 CHAPTER 7, was correctly and truly scientifically isolated prior to the date of the Coronavirus Act 2020 CHAPTER 7 which is shown as dated 25th March 2020? This request is formally made under the Freedom of Information Act 2000 in this publication and in the letter dated 3rd October 2022 included in the Appendices of this book.

Further, there was never a "pandemic"

It is clear that Covid19 has much the same fatality rate (c. 0.14% of population) as the Common Flu which we have annually, clearly demonstrate that the **UK "Covid19" Mandates were not reasonable, proportionate, appropriate, nor necessary.** We do not globally lockdown the entire global Capitalist system for the Common Flu every year so why did we do it for "Covid19" which is no more harmful? It cannot be lawful, in any country that has any pretence for respect for law and order, for an enormous program of "vaccines" and "vaccination" of entire populations including children can be implemented and based on "laws" and "mandates" that are **not reasonable, proportionate, appropriate, nor necessary.**

Further, there was **NO informed consent** to take the "vaccines" because the recipients of the injections had no knowledge of the content of the "vaccines" (nor did the idiots who were "vaccinating" them, nor did the idiots who authorized this monstrous nonsense: Hancock, Johnson, Sajid, Zahawi, GMC, NHS et al) nor full information of their potential adverse effects nor were the population properly informed that they were not truly "vaccines" but Messenger RNA (single stranded RNA) mRNA treatments. If the world's population had been informed of the contents of these "vaccines" – they would have run a mile!

Furthermore, the global population was not informed that these "vaccines" had not undergone full clinical trials – a process that usually takes 7 to 10 years. The "vaccines" were rushed to the market under the title of "experimental". Consequently, the world's population was, in reality, **The Experiment**. The World's population was in fact, **"Sars-Cov-2"/"Covid19" Human Guinea Pigs, without the knowledge of what they were getting themselves into nor giving the required informed consent for having their bodies injected with poison !**

This reminds one of Joseph Mengeles "Angel of Death" the infamous Nazi "doctor" who performed medical experiments at the **Auschwitz death camps**, but much, much worse – **in this case the entire global population was the experiment.**

A further tragedy was that the world's populations were not informed that the "vaccines", supposedly created to solve the problem of a "virus", that was not a virus! **The "virus" was not a virus it was a Bioweapon/Chemical Weapon containing HIV spike proteins**. As confirmed by Dr Poorminha Wagh previously quoted and again below:

Dr Poornima Wagh, Researcher, 2 PhDs in Virology and Immunology, Santa Barbara, CA, USA

Quote:

***"How do you find HIV spike proteins in a 'NOVEL' virus genome? You don't, it's called FRAUD"* [What has been called, by WHO etc. "Sars-Cov-2" IS NOT a virus!]**

We can clearly observe from the facts above, listed below, that the UK Coronavirus Act 2020 is most possibly unlawful and would not stand up to close scrutiny. Facts:

1. "SarsCov2" has not been isolated, therefore identified, so how can you legislate for it!? Clearly demonstrated above.
2. Alberta law case, Canada; resulting in the UK Crown and Privy Counsel and its advisors not being able to provide proof of isolation of "SarsCov2"
3. "SarsCov2" has not been isolated - "NOT FOUND" in world-wide search
4. There was never a "pandemic" (0.14% fatality for "SarsCov2" – same as flu)
5. There was no informed consent – Big Pharma hid the truth of "virus" & "vaccines"
6. "SarsCov2" was not a "virus" but a Bioweapon/Chemical Weapon – unlawful
7. Laws must be **reasonable, proportionate, appropriate, and necessary.**

CORONA ACCOUNTABILITY (Covid19) 2022 considers that The UK Coronavirus Act 2020 is most possibly unlawful, illegal and that it should be subject to review. Reports inform that unlawful acts and have been propagated in recent years by the UK Government.

Johnson's suspension of parliament unlawful, Supreme Court rules

'The [UK] Supreme Court has ruled that Boris Johnson's [Prime Minister] advice to the Queen that parliament should be prorogued for five weeks at the height of the Brexit crisis was unlawful.

The unanimous judgment from 11 justices on the UK's highest court followed an emergency three-day hearing last week that exposed fundamental legal differences over interpreting the country's unwritten constitution.

The momentous decision was read out by Lady Hale, president of the Supreme Court. Unusually, none of the parties were provided with advance copies of the judgment due to its sensitivity.'

Ref: https://www.theguardian.com/law/2019/sep/24/boris-johnsons-suspension-of-parliament-unlawful-supreme-court-rules-prorogue

Other examples of the disregard for laws, rules and regulations by the UK Boris Johnson Government in recent years:

1. The PM flat refurbishment
2. Owen Paterson lobbying scandal
3. 'Partygate'
4. Pincher misconduct allegations

Ref: https://www.cnn.com/2022/07/06/uk/boris-johnson-scandals-intl/index.html

Furthermore:

'Johnson's Lies Worked for Years, Until They Didn't'

'People have known that Boris Johnson lies for 30 years,' the writer and academic Rory Stewart, a former Conservative member of Parliament ***'He's probably the best liar we've ever had as a prime minister. He knows a hundred different ways to lie.'***

Ref: https://www.nytimes.com/2022/07/08/world/europe/boris-johnson-lies-britain-parliament.html

In Italy we have:

Vittorio Sgarbi - Italian Chamber of Deputies Exclamation

The excuse for murdering millions of people [Chapter 11] with these injections is that they supposedly prevent people from dying of "Covid". The reality is however that the so-called number of "Covid" deaths is the **greatest lie in history**. **Worldwide it was revealed that over 95% of all "Covid" deaths, were deaths from other causes.**

The Italian politician Vittorio Sgarbi exclaimed in the Italian Chamber of Deputies:

'Let's not make this the chamber of lies. Don't lie! Tell the truth. Don't say there's 25,000 dead. It's not true. Don't use the dead for rhetoric and terrorism. Figures from the Higher Institute of Health say 96.3% died of other diseases.'

An Undertaker Witnesses UK Government Crimes

Ref: https://stopworldcontrol.com/director/

One very revealing eyewitness account comes from a **funeral director from the UK, John O'Looney.** For 10 years he was part of one of the largest funeral companies in the United Kingdom, he worked with the BBC to document the "pandemic" and worked with a government "pandemic" official. He is connected to 45 other funeral directors and has therefore a clear overview of what is going on. **What he discloses is shocking.**

First of all, he testifies that neither he nor any of the other funeral directors saw an increase in deaths during the so-called "pandemic".

During March 2020 however, John O'Looney was suddenly called night after night, for three weeks, specifically to care homes. **All who died were labelled as "Covid". He never saw a doctor in attendance, nor a "Covid" test once. At the same time, there was a 1,000% increase in purchases of Midazolam. A nurse told him how they were instructed to administer lethal doses of this drug to the elderly, to mass exterminate them. These high numbers of deaths were then used to promote the narrative of a "covid pandemic". He was also approached by a government "pandemic" official, who told him they had to label each death as "Covid". People run over by cars, heart attacks, cancer patients, it didn't matter what killed them, they all had to be labelled as "Covid" deaths.**

It is important to note here that there are Reports of Matt Hancock and others being prosecuted for the misuse of Midazolam for "end of life care" in Care Homes. This confirms the report above by John O'Looney!

The allegations are against the Matt Hancock and other Government officials for mass murder!

'Next week, after a calculated delay between the start of "COVID-1984" and the present day, the TGBMS Class Action to end institutionalised mortgage fraud and signature forgery in the UK will suddenly lurch forward once again; along with the Private Criminal Prosecution of the Midazolam Murderers, from the men and women in white and blue coats, all the way up to **[Matt]** *Hancock et al, in the murderous supply chain for the deadly drug that has been and continues to be used to euthanize people by government policy.'*

- posted on 24th May 2022 by The Bernician, reference below:

Ref: https://www.thebernician.net/tgbms-class-action-midazolam-murders-pcp-move-forward/

To return to John O'Looney's evidence:

Ref: https://stopworldcontrol.com/director/

Once the government started mass "vaccinating" the British population, John O'Looney says the <u>deaths skyrocketed</u>.

'I've never seen anything like it, as a funeral director for fifteen years. And it began exactly when they began putting* [Covid19"]** ***needles in their arms. I've never seen a death rate like that again. It was awful, awful. <u>Those were pandemic numbers, but it was only after they started "vaccinating", never before that point.</u>'

John explains that most vaccine deaths were [unlawfully] labelled "Covid" deaths.

John O'Looney quote:

'Every funeral director with an ounce of honesty will tell you that all those who are dying all around us are <u>"vaccine" recipients</u>. <u>There is no "covid" pandemic and I am living proof of that</u>. <u>It's all designed to make you take the "vaccine"</u>. In my network of funeral directors, not a single child has died of "covid". So, there is no reason whatsoever to put these gene therapies into children. <u>Here we have a depopulation agenda. It's the "vaccines" that are killing the people, and I am seeing that first-hand as a funeral director</u>.'

In a video interview John O'Looney gives even more shocking revelations about the **numbers of deaths of children because of these deadly "vaccines"**.

He further states that a specialist Gas/Oil Rig Engineering Human Resources Company were asked to mass recruit new unvaccinated staff to replace the "vaccinated" staff because the "vaccinated" staff were <u>expected to die within the next three years</u>! Video entitled 'Live with John O'Looney' - Broadcast 29th August 2022

Ref: https://www.lauralynn.tv/search?updated-max=2022-09-01T15:27:00-07:00&max-results=5

"Covid19" Fraud Summary

1. Health care workers are paid or pressured to register all patients as "Covid"
2. The hundreds of millions of flu cases every year are now all "Covid"
3. A forensic German coroner examined 140 "corona" fatalities and said they all died of other causes and there is no killer "virus"
4. Doctors get hidden messages requiring them to register dying patients as "Covid" deaths
5. A network of 20 hospitals is caught increasing covid numbers to create fear

6. Innumerable people worldwide are outraged because they were incorrectly registered as "Covid"
7. Funeral directors admit they see false "Covid" registrations all the time
8. CNN technical director Chester confessed they inflate "Covid" numbers because 'fear sells'
9. An African government official is seen in a Zoom call discussing how to ramp up "Covid" numbers, in order to continue the lockdowns
10. The Italian politician Vittorio is infuriated because he sees how the chamber is lying: only a small percentage died of "Covid"!
11. A funeral director witnesses the murder of thousands of elderly, to create so-called "Covid" deaths
12. He and dozens of other funeral directors were instructed by the British government to label every death as "Covid"
13. Once the "vaccinations" started, these funeral directors witnessed an unprecedented explosion of deaths

Ref: https://stopworldcontrol.com/director/

Treatments for "Covid19" already available worldwide

There were treatments for this "virus" available and ready to use immediately!

Ref: https://stopworldcontrol.com/downloads/en/vaccines/vaccinereport.pdf

From the very start of this worldwide "health crisis", there were many prominent scientists and medical doctors who exclaimed how they were successfully treating many thousands of "Covid" patients using existing drugs that are known for their safety and efficacy. There is for example the world-famous French professor Didier Raoult, director of one of the largest research groups in infectious diseases and microbiology. He is the most cited microbiologist in Europe according to ISI and has trained more than 457 foreign scientists in his lab since 1998 with more than 1950 articles referred in ISI or Pubmed and is considered the world's foremost expert on infectious diseases. **Professor Raoult started treating "Covid" patients with a medicine that has been around for <u>over sixty years</u> and is famous for its safety and efficiency in defeating coronaviruses: hydroxychloroquine.**

Professor Raoult treated over four thousand patients with hydroxychloroquine + azithromycin and virtually all of them recovered, except for a handful of very elderly who already had several morbidities.

More details of these available treatments are dealt with in Chapter 3 and Chapter 15.

With several options to successfully treat COVID-19, why is there still such an outcry for a "vaccine"? And why is the majority of the population not even aware of the available treatments? The answer is shocking and shows once more what is going on in our world...

All over the world physicians who were successfully treating "Covid" patients [without "vaccines"], encountered the unthinkable: they were intimidated and shut down by the government.

This MUST be unlawful!! These world physicians were unlawfully obliged to break their Hippocratic Oath!!

America's Frontline Doctors informed the world about the safe and effective cures for covid, during their first White Coat Summit in 2020. This broadcast was viewed over twenty million times in a few hours, but then they were shut down all across the board: Facebook, YouTube, Twitter, and even their website was taken down by Squarespace.

Dr. David Brownstein from Michigan, a leading holistic practitioner, had successfully treated over 120 "Covid" patients, but his entire medical blog was removed. Dr. Rob Elens who successfully treated all his "Covid" patients in the Netherlands was **threatened by the government that he would lose his license if he continued treating these people**. Dr. Joseph Mercola, a leading voice worldwide in healthy living, published information on how to treat "Covid" and was forced to delete his content after Google had already banned him. Professor Raoult, who is one of the most respected scientists in the world, is suddenly slandered all over the internet. Dr. Zelenko who successfully treated over 6,000 patients, among whom two presidents and the Israeli health minister, is also bashed all over the web, and even had to leave his community because of the backlash.

The biophysicist Andreas Kalcker was de-platformed from all major social media, his book was removed from Amazon and even his scientific account on ResearchGate was deleted.

For the first time since Stalin's Programs, we see Medico-Totalitarianism on a global scale that the Master Dictator Stalin would have been jealous of!

All these, together with those in Chapter 3 are just a few of the examples of physicians and scientists who successfully treated "Covid" patients without using the "vaccines", **who faced massive opposition**.

Never before in the history of mankind has it occurred that a working and safe drug for an illness has been kept from the world, through such a global, internationally coordinated, effort.

People are not supposed to recover from "Covid", because the world population needs to be scared into accepting this potentially lethal injection.

It is clear, that the deliberate oppression of perfectly safe, effective and well tested treatments for "Covid19" by Governments and others in authority can have NO legitimacy in LAW!

To repeat:

It is clear, that the deliberate oppression of perfectly safe, effective and well tested treatments for "Covid19" by Governments and others in authority can have NO legitimacy in LAW!

It is particularly obnoxious that these perfectly safe, effective and well tested treatments for "Covid19" should be deliberately usurped by Governments and others in authority so that preference would be given to untested, un-trialled, experimental "vaccines" that did not work, were completely useless in their application for solving "Covid" and were, in truth, dangerous Bioweapons/Chemical Weapons enforced upon an unsuspecting global population for the surreptitious purpose of killing that population!

Why would the "elite" [Evil300] desire a growing population of homo sapiens and all the social/economic/human problems that go with that growing population; soon to be 10Bn and rising, when a lot of their economic/work efforts will be replaced by Robots/AI/Machine Learning/Quantum Computing/Big Data etc by 2050 or thereabouts.

A drop of 3-in-one oil (light viscosity) on a robot's arm is much cheaper than amputating a human limb when the human operative fails to operate efficiently.

CHAPTER 14

WHY THE THIRTEEN CONFIDENCE TRICKS TOOK PLACE & THE DAMAGE CAUSED

'NEW WORLD ORDER'

For
'NEW WORLD ORDER'
read

'Post-Industrial, Quasi-feudal, Dystopian Mass-Slave Totalitarianism'

Australia, one of the fiercest of 'Lockdown' totalitarianisms, no longer hides what is going on!

Ref: https://stopworldcontrol.com/downloads/en/vaccines/vaccinereport.pdf

For decades the tyrannical system of worldwide oppression and control, called the **New World Order**, was labelled a 'conspiracy theory'. But as it is with many so-called 'conspiracy theories', after some time they prove to be more than theories – they are facts! We understand that the term 'Conspiracy Theory' was originated by the CIA USA using that tired, very dull, pseudo-legal technique, that if you cannot refute the evidence, then try to denigrate the witness themselves by character assassination etc. In this case the CIA tried to denigrate the evidence by calling it a "Conspiracy".

In Australia, the health officials no longer hide their agenda, and have been calling their "Covid" tyranny the **'New World Order.'** This is what the Chief Health Officer of New South Wales, Kerry Gai Chant, said during a public broadcast:

'We will be looking at what contact tracing looks like in the New World Order. Yes, it will be pubs and clubs and other things if we have a positive case there.'

Brad Hazard, the Australian Health Minister, said the following words:

'That's just the way it is. We have got to accept that this is the New World Order'.

An Australian news reporter announced new restrictions with the following words:

'Also, the New World Order that will come into force at 12pm, at midnight tonight, new restrictions on various businesses.'

Another Australian news broadcast, said it like this:

'The New World Order, our army comes marching in, partnering with police, to help enforce the country's tough new quarantine laws.'

The day that the new restrictions came into place, the news reporter said:

'Today is the first full day of the New World Order. Outdoor gatherings are limited to two people. Exercise is allowed but no further than a 10km radius from your home. Browsing in shops is not permitted. Only one person per household may leave to do essential shopping. And from tomorrow funerals are limited to ten people.'

What is the excuse for this inhumane tyranny?

14 supposed "Covid" deaths during the first half of 2021! While in 2017 over four thousand people died in Australia from influenza and pneumonia.

Only an idiot would believe that this has anything to do with health.

Furthermore, only an idiot would parrot the garbage, "*New World Order*" they are given to parrot by puppets of bigger idiots. These clowns would not know a "New World Order" from a New World Oven! This "*New World Order*" garbage must be the biggest Intellectual Insult in the entire history of homo sapiens.

Similar antics, to varying degrees, took place all over the world. Another of the fiercest 'Lockdowns' in the 'Western World' was Canada. This caused the largest display of rebellion against this tyranny by the Canadian Truckers, who presented to the world a coherent response to that child and puppet of The Privy Council, Justin Trudeau. Their brave resistance was a beacon of light and hope to the world, in its darkest hour.

Australia Tyranny Exposed

However, in Australia, good people are exposing this disgusting, dystopian tyranny!

Covid Inquiry 2.0 by Senator Malcolm Roberts, Australia - 16th August 2022

Referring to those responsible for the "SarCov2" "Covid19" "pandemic" lies:

'We will hound you down!'

'It has become clear, the people of this country* [Australia] *and globally have been steamrollered. It is also clear that it has been coordinated globally. It is also clear that it has been integrated not just over 6 months, not just over 2 ½ years, but it has been planned over decades. The changes to legislation in this country were done so that they could control doctors and the people.

People are awakening and its thanks to Dr Altman and all the presenters here today. ***We know that this* ["SarCov2" "Covid19" "pandemic"] IS ALL BULLSHIT and we've been HAD.**

But we are going to hound you down. – you people who are guilty.

We will hound you down and hold you accountable and we will expose you globally, so that the people of Australia look forward to the future, because I love my kids and I'm looking forward to my grandkids.

We are going to save this country. Thank you.'

Ref 1: https://twitter.com/EleonoreNemethM/status/1560878573925404672 20th Aug. 2022

Ref 2: https://rumble.com/v1g95tl-covid-inquiry-2.0.html 16th August 2022

Who is Ultimately Responsible?

Ref: https://stopworldcontrol.com/downloads/en/vaccines/vaccinereport.pdf

Who exactly are these psychopathic criminals? Do we have some of their names and whereabouts? How do they operate and what can we do to stop them? An important part of the answer is given in the magnificent documentary **'MONOPOLY'**, can be viewed on timgielen.com, see reference below:

Ref: https://www.timgielen.com/videos/ [Tim Gielen]

The Families of Great Power

TIM GIELDEN for MONOPOLY reveals in great detail, with all the evidence on screen, how virtually everything in our world is owned by the same people, and it shows what they are planning for humanity.

In the documentary 'MONOPOLY', very relevant to the "Covid19" crisis in 2020, **Marc van Ranst a leading Belgian** "virologist" gives a shocking and cynical presentation on 22nd January 2019 to delegates at **'Chatham House'** **'The Royal Institute for International Affairs' in London** about his experience in Belgium during the Swine Flu in 2009.

At **'The Royal Institute for International Affairs' in London,** the reigning sovereign serves as **Patron** of the institute - **Her Majesty Queen Elizabeth II has been Patron since her accession to the throne in 1952. We trust that Her Majesty was not present when van Ranst described his methods for fear mongering, out of context mortality rates and media manipulation.**

He describes his methods for fear mongering, out of context mortality rates and media manipulation. How he imposed the "vaccines" on a frightened Belgian population – "vaccines" produced by the companies he worked for.

To quote this Deontological Ethicist of "Genius":

'You get complete **[media]** ***coverage so that they*** **[the media]** ***do not search for alternatives.'*** [He used extensive media propaganda methodology.]

'I misused the fact the top football soccer players in Belgium against all agreements inappropriately made their soccer players priority people. So, I said I can use that because if the population really believes that for this "vaccine" that even these soccer players would dishonestly get their "vaccine". I said OK, I can play with that. So, I made a big fuss about this.' [in the media]

'This van Ranst is raving mad [in the media] ***but it worked.'***

For those with stomach reflexes strong enough for this crass vulgarity, this van Ranst presentation can be viewed at mins:secs 42:46 – 47:23 on video:

Ref: https://www.timgielen.com/videos/

Because these superrich entities own everything, it's a piece of cake for them to control the world. They own Apple, Facebook, Twitter, Google, Facebook, and the rest of Big Tech, all the major news media, the entire travel industry, the whole food industry, the banks, the clothing industry, and so on.

By strategically buying everything, they have gained an unrivalled monopoly worldwide. Something Julius Caesar could only dream of... They also own the entire health industry, which allows them to tell hospitals around the world what to do and what not to do. They have positioned their political puppets in governments around the world through election fraud, bribery and blackmailing. Once we understand this, we can see how they are able to impose tyranny all over the world.

It would take too long to name all the involved individual entities, but I will reveal a few, that are at the heart of this network. In Italy there are for example 13 Italian families or bloodlines, called the 'Black Nobility', The 'mafia on steroids'. These families, along with other similar dynasties from other regions of the earth, consider themselves to be superior over the rest of humanity. They look upon regular folks as 'livestock', 'cattle', 'useless eaters' etc. That is literally how they write about you in their literature.

They believe that it's their destiny to rule over humanity, who are to become their slaves

[This has been the situation, particularly in Europe since the introduction of Feudalism in the 11th Century. Feudalism predated the nation-state; at that time, there was no organised state. The 'capital' was heritable land and property; the heritable nature of the land and property was very important to the social fabric of feudal society, since position and wealth accrued in the present was safeguarded for the future by the inheritable system that passed wealth from the present generation to the eldest son of the next. As with all other forms of 'capitalism', the key to the success of the system was a **vertical hierarchical structure of ownership by the owners and obedience to those who did own, by those who did not.** Those at the top of the structure owned, those in the middle owned little or leased, and **those at the bottom owned nothing other than their capacity for obedience and reproduction.**

The feudal system, in essence, consisted of fiefdoms of heritable land, property or rights owned by the nobility. The land owned by the nobility was inheritable by the nobleman's eldest son. The fief usually consisted of land and the **peasants laboured to cultivate it**. They were bound to the land in rented accommodation owned by the Baron, Earl or Lord.

Any disobedience and the land labourer and his family was potentially without work and without a home.]

Ref:

SAVE YOURSELF SAVE US ALL
How We Can Survive Happily into the 22nd Century
The Unique Post Covid-19 Opportunity for All Humankind
(Chapter 1)
by
Lawrence Wolfe-Xavier

[Publ. 2021]

Ref: https://saveyourselfsaveusall.co.uk/

To repeat:

They believe that it's their destiny to rule over humanity, who are to become their slaves.

Ref: https://stopworldcontrol.com/downloads/en/vaccines/vaccinereport.pdf

These families are organized in a pyramidal hierarchy, [as since 11th Century Feudalism above] where ultimately everyone answers to the same puppet masters at the top [in Feudalism the peak of the pyramid was the King].

Today the key to their power is secrecy, so nobody can touch them. **That's why the real leaders always stay in the shadows.** The world population only sees puppets that operate on the visible stage of the world scene, like mind-programmed politicians, perverted Hollywood celebrities, industrial leaders, media personalities, etc. **Some better-known puppets are Klaus Schwab WEF, Bill Gates, George Soros, the Clintons, Bush and Morgan families, etc.** Although they are all individually very rich and powerful, they are submitted to entities that are higher up in the hierarchy, but who make sure they - the highest entities, stay out of the picture. ***Secrecy is their strength.***

However, they are easily known to those who trouble to seek them. It is estimated that the top of this tyrannical pyramid consists of c. Thirteen Families or so with complete global reach, with others subordinate under them. The top thirteen bully their underlings.

The Front Men & Front Organisations for The Families

World Health Organization 'WHO'

One of their strategies is to set up public 'global' organizations, which are their visible platforms to work out their agenda. One of these has become very prominent during this organized "pandemic" and is called the World Health Organization 'WHO', which is mostly financed by **Bill Gates, a key puppet of this criminal network**. The WHO is dictating to all of humanity - think about this! - what we can or cannot do when it comes to our health our bodies, that are sovereign to each person!

Nobody elected the World Health Organization and nobody wants them to be around, to bully every physician, nurse, and health practitioner into blind obedience.

The WHO forces the entire world into unquestioning submission to their tyrannical 'guidelines', that are more often anti-scientific than based on proper science.

The WHO for example told the entire world to use the PCR test to discover "Covid" cases, while this test cannot discern between different types of pathogens and produces up to 93% of false positives. This flawed test is the main tool to tell the world there is a pandemic, while **no medical device in history has ever been so unreliable**. Yet this anti-scientific protocol is imposed on the entire world, to promote the illusion of a global "pandemic", which is mainly based on false positives. The hundreds of millions of so-called "Covid cases" are nothing but false positives, resulting from a fatally flawed test. **The actual "virus" "Sars-Cov-2" has never been isolated and purified; therefore, it is impossible to test for it. It's a scam of astronomical proportions.**

That's an example of how a 'world organization' is used to roll out the agenda of submitting humanity to tyranny, in the name of 'protecting your health'.

United Nations 'UN'

A similar organization is the **United Nations**, which portrays itself as the so-called 'peacekeeper' of this world. Their agenda is however to submit all of humanity to a one-world government. The U.N. works closely with the **European Union** and **NATO**, which are similar carousels for the criminal families to wipe out the independence of the sovereign nations and set up a one-world government.

World Economic Forum 'WEF'

Another public player is the **World Economic Forum**, founded by **Klaus Schwab,** sponsored by Henry Kissinger, perhaps the world's first true globalist, in the early 1970s. The World Economic Forum presents itself as a think tank for the rich and powerful of the world, where they 'seek solutions for the world's problems'. Their magic term is 'sustainable development' which claims to ensure a better future for our world. Together with the U.N., they developed the so-called Agenda 2030, which claims to offer the ultimate solution for a more sustainable world.

For 'sustainable development' see definition below:

Ref: **Peter Wood, Economist**

What is "Sustainable Development"?

Grand Jury Day 5 Economical and Financial Destruction:

Sustainable Development aka Technocracy	**Capitalism Free Market Economy**
Scientific management of resources and consumption	Price-based free market economy determined by supply and demand
FinTech is underlying financial system (blockchain, digital currencies, total surveillance)	Currency based capital is underlying financial system
No private property. Resources held in global common trust	Ownership and use of private property is fundamental right
No privacy allowed	Privacy is fundamental right

In reality, this means nothing less than seizing all rights, freedoms and properties from the entire world population and bringing it all in the hands of the superrich.

As mentioned above, **Klaus Schwab WEF, Bill Gates, George Soros, the Clintons, the Bush family, the Morgan family are front men for the real Evil300 'leaders' who stay in the shadows.**

The World Bank & The Finance System

Then there is the banking imperium, which controls all the money supply in the world. Their job is to bring about a cashless society where only those who are digitally connected to the system of surveillance and slavery, will still have access to finances. **The Nigerian government has been paid handsomely by them, to reserve banking services strictly for the "vaccinated"**, an example that will soon be followed by other countries. A leading entity in the banking imperium is the notorious **Rothschild family**. **They own the central banks in 165 nations, thus controlling the money flow in most of the world**. Since ancient times this family has dedicated itself to the worship of the darkest of all forces. **Another well-known, equally dark family are the Rockefellers. They published the 'Scenario of the Future' in 2010, in which they described the current pandemic in great detail, with the desired outcome of establishing a new world of domination and control.**

Entities like the Rockefeller Institute present themselves as protectors of humanity, but behind this humanitarian mask there is a gruesome face of lust for power and control.

"Christianity"

Already mentioned was the Black Nobility from Italy. Their most effective strategy has been to hide behind the beautiful face of Christianity, as they established the Vatican in Rome, as the 'centre of Roman Catholicism'. Behind the monumental architecture of the majestic cathedrals, there however lurks a world so dark and perverse, that no normal human being could ever comprehend it. The recent exposure of organized, systematic child abuse in this religious stronghold is only the tiniest tip of an iceberg so deep, that it would traumatize most of us, if we knew what is going on there. Make no mistake: there are also good religious people in the Vatican, who are opposing the criminal activities.

For example, archbishop Carlo Maria Vigano, has been speaking out against what he calls the 'Deep Church', comparing it to the 'Deep State'.

The Vatican is located inside Vatican City, which is a sovereign state independent from Italy, where no Italian law has any authority. Because they are not submitted to the laws of any land, not even Italy that surrounds them, they are able to commit any crime they want. Similar sovereign states inside the nations are 'The City of London Corporation' (an independent state within London that evades all British laws but controls the British government), 'Washington D.C.' (or the District of Columbia, which is a sovereign state inside the United States, that rules over the American people). The criminal families have set up these untouchable 'states within nations' from where they operate.

Vatican City is the most important of them all, and it is here that the highest puppet masters have their seat.

We all know the White Pope, a role that is currently played by Pope Francis. His job is to control the worldwide Roman Catholic faith community and steer them towards the New World Order. In several public messages he calls all believers to get vaccinated and goes on to proclaim the **New World Order** as the only solution to the world's problems. Here are some of his statements:

'We can heal injustice by building **a new world order** ... The path to humanity's salvation passes through the creation of **a new model** of development ... take care of the Earth, with **radical personal and political choices, ... without an overall vision** there will be no future ... we must bring an end to **short-sighted nationalism** ...'

Besides the **White Pope**, there is also a lesser-known **Black Pope** who has far more power, but who works more behind the scenes. The Black Pope however is still submitted to one who sits on a higher throne: the **Grey Pope**. This supreme puppet master operates entirely in the shadows, from where he yields enormous power over the world. If you want to understand how all this originated historically, you have to research the dark spiritual origins of the Jesuits.

We must understand that this criminal network is highly "spiritual" in nature, and all who are at the top, are involved in dark ancient "spiritual" practices.

We see this with Klaus Schwab, [WEF] who uses eloquent rhetoric to bewitch the minds of his worldwide audience and convince them that the noblest of all causes is to make sure that every human on earth will think and feel the exact same way. *'Lift humanity into a collective consciousness.'* Quote.

The way he presents this stark raving mad plan, is however so cunning that most people would give him a standing ovation, after hearing his speech. The same we see with the White Pope, who speaks beautifully about caring for the poor, ending injustice, saving the

Earth, and other noble causes, [However he has not done much for the 80% of the world, it would appear, who still live off less than 10US$ per day - simply google it!] while in fact he simply says: 'The whole world needs to be enslaved to a one world government, where nobody will have a voice, rights, freedoms, possessions, identity or privacy.' It's the same kind of hypnosis they use to impose the "vaccine" mandates: 'The world is attacked by a deadly disease, but we have a wonderful solution: lifesaving "vaccines". Hurray!' That these wonderful "vaccines" contain ostensibly living creatures with tentacles, self-assembling nanobots, highly toxic substances – spike proteins, graphene oxide etc, and that millions are killed by them, or harmed by them, is of course not mentioned.

It's all about hypnotizing humanity using refined forms of hypocrisy and deception.

Another way these criminals operate is by organizing themselves in so-called **secret societies**, to establish their hidden influence in every nation. Apart from the completely hidden societies, there are also more public cults, such as **Freemasonry**. This is one of the better-known "spiritual" organizations, used to influence local authorities in virtually every town of every nation. They attract people in authority, claiming to be an innocent organization that wants to help humanity. Only when members climb to the higher levels of Freemasonry, do they discover the truth. By then it is too late – you are enslaved in the cult with little or no escape.

Freemasonry focuses on making influential people in every community their members, so they can use them for the outworking of their plans. Google whistle-blower Zach Vorhies stated that in 2016 **Google laid out their plans to program humanity in a revealing location: the San Francisco Freemasonry Headquarters**. There Google informed their staff about the company strategy: **mould the mind of mankind**. That illustrates how Freemasonry plays a central role in this worldwide globalist agenda.

Military Secret Services

The many secret societies work closely with the secret services of the nations, for example the **CIA** and **FBI** in America. Entities that on the surface fight crime, but in reality, are among the worst of all criminal organizations. The renowned German journalist Udo Ulfkotte, who was murdered for his confessions, admitted a few years ago that journalists all over the world are paid by secret services, secret societies, government agencies, billionaires, etc. to always lie and never tell the truth to the public.

His important testimony can be seen in the documentary **'BUSTED'** on StopWorldControl.com. It is because of the confessions of this brave journalist - who was editor of one of Europe's largest newspapers - that a major awakening is going on in Germany. His book opened the eyes of the German population, who are now a major force against the "New World Order".

'BUSTED' Ref: https://stopworldcontrol.com/media/

Is there any hope for humanity? YES.

This subject is dealt with in chapters 15, 16, 17, 20 and 21.

CHAPTER 15

HOW TO RETURN TO YOUR PRE-"COVID19" GOOD HEALTH- "COVID19" TREATMENTS

There was Never Any Need for the DEADLY "VACCINES"

The World is Awakening to this Evil

Good news is that there has been a lot of infighting in this criminal network, causing it to fall apart in several camps, camps that all compete for world domination. May this confusion among them increase, as they fall into their own pits, and their plans fail miserably.

Much more can be said about all of this, as many books have been written about this criminal network, by researchers who often dedicated their entire lives to expose them. If you want to learn more, you can find a wealth of quality information compiled by some excellent researchers on the Dutch website **Ellaster.nl**. Use Google translate to read the articles in your own language if different from the original:

Ref: https://www.ellaster.nl/category/val-van-cabal/cabal/

Is there any hope for humanity? YES! YES! YES!

Although we are witnessing the greatest criminal operation since the birth of our 'modern' world of the last 2,000 years, something entirely different is also happening. Hundreds of millions of people are waking up from the deep sleep of ignorance and deception, and they are letting out a roar of truth, all over the world. In every nation organisations of medical doctors, lawyers, scientists, and all kinds of professionals are being established, to fight for freedom. They consist of tens of thousands of educated, influential and passionate professionals who are determined to stop this diabolical scheme. Brand new media platforms are being born, that grow every day in influence. They are not owned by the criminal cartel but work from a heart that wants to defend humanity against the onslaught of destructive fake news media that is operated by the cabal.

Ref: https://stopworldcontrol.com/downloads/en/vaccines/vaccinereport.pdf

On top of that, increasingly large numbers of health care workers are refusing the "vaccine" mandates. In Canada 35,000 medical professionals protested against the "vaccines". In New York 83,000 health care workers refuse the toxic injections. Overall, in the U.S. 58% of all physicians is not taking the dangerous shots. Also, among law enforcement and fire fighters there is increasing protest against the "vaccine" mandates. In California 50% of all law enforcement stands up against these criminal mandates. In Australia, one of the most severely and most repressively 'locked down' countries in the world, Senator Malcolm Roberts was vehemently clear in his response to this criminality at the **"Covid" Inquiry 2.0**:

"Covid" Inquiry 2.0 by Senator Malcolm Roberts, Australia - 16th August 2022

Referring to those responsible for the "SarCov2" "Covid19" "pandemic" lies:

'We will hound you down!'

'*It has become clear, the people of this country* [Australia] *and globally have been steamrollered. It is also clear that it has been coordinated globally. It is also clear that it has been integrated not just over 6 months, not just over 2 ½ years, but it has been planned over decades. The changes to legislation in this country were done so that they could control doctors and the people.*

People are awakening and its thanks to Dr Altman and all the presenters here today. ***We know that this*** **["SarCov2" "Covid19" "pandemic"] IS ALL BULLSHIT and we've been HAD.**

But we are going to hound you down. – you people who are guilty. ***We will hound you down and hold you accountable and we will expose you globally, so that the people of Australia look forward to the future, because I love my kids and I'm looking forward to my grandkids.***

We are going to save this country. Thank you.'

Ref 1: https://twitter.com/EleonoreNemethM/status/1560878573925404672 20th Aug. 2022

Ref 2: https://rumble.com/v1g95tl-covid-inquiry-2.0.html 16th August 2022

These are just a few examples of the mass non-compliance in nations around the world.

This resistance is about to explode even furthermore worldwide, as the truth about these injections is spreading far and wide, despite all the attempts from the ***criminal "vaccine" cartel*** - which includes Big Tech, Big Pharma, government agencies, news media, etc. - to suppress this information.

Stop World Control

StopWorldControl.com is to launch a world map, that will show hundreds of organizations in nations around the world who are resisting this criminal operation. They represent hundreds of millions of people who refuse to become slaves of criminals. Among them are large numbers of physicians, scientists, academics, lawyers, entrepreneurs, politicians, etc.

Ref: https://stopworldcontrol.com/

There is an unprecedented and unstoppable awakening going on, that will only increase in the near future.

Stop World Control is investigating proposed solutions to detox from the "Covid" "vaccines". We have found several options that are promising, and we hope to release a Vaccine Detox Guide soon. Sadly, not every damage done by the mRNA shots will be able to be undone, like the altering of the DNA. That is a switch that cannot be reversed [according to current research]. There are however methods to get rid of the nanotech in your body, kill the living organisms that are being injected, remove the spike proteins, etc. As vaccinations continue, and different pathogens will be released, we will keep researching for any new solutions that will become available. Sign up for the emails of Stop World Control to stay updated on this research. If you know of working solutions to detox from these injections, please email us at network@stopworldcontrol.com

Patient Information assisting in dealing with "Covid19" is available on the following websites:

www.CovidPatientGuide.com – Downloadable Physician List & Guide to Home-Based COVID Treatment

www.C19Protocols.com – Two Post Vaccination Protocols, 13 Early Treatment Protocols, 4 Long Covid Protocols

www.TheCovidRemedy.com General Advice and Guidance on "Covid" Introductory Video banned by Social Media Giants

www.FlemingMethod.com/best-available-published-evidence General Advice and Guidance on "Covid"

www.StopWorldControl.com/cures Good background information. Cures used are detailed in this book.

World Leading Scientists and Medics offering "Covid19" Remedies

Ref: **www.StopWorldControl.com/cures**

Professor Didier Raoult, MD, PhD - The world's leading expert in infectious diseases – developed cure number one:

Cure No 1: Hydroxychloroquine (HCQ) + Zinc

Dr. Simone Gold, MD, JD, FABEM - who was the spokesperson for over 600 medical doctors in America, tweeted that countries administering Hydroxychloroquine 'HCQ' have a 79.1% lower mortality rate. When HCQ is given in early stages of "COVID-19", there is a 100% survival rate.

Dr. Rob Elens, MD - In The Netherlands Dr. Rob Elens gave all his "Covid" patients hydroxychloroquine combined with zinc and saw a 100% recovery rate in an average of four days. Nobody needed to be hospitalized. Along with 2,700+ (!) other medical professionals he sent a letter to the Dutch government, to defend hydroxychloroquine and ask them to include it into the standard protocol. Dr Elens and other Dutch medical doctors set up a "Covid19" Self -Care website 'COVID-19 Self Care' website, with information on how to prevent and overcome "COVID-19", using HCQ and zinc. It is available in English.

Ref: https://zelfzorgcovid19.nl/

Dr Vladimir Zelenko (now deceased) Helped 1000+ Covid Patients Recover.

In New York the Family Practitioner Dr. Vladimir Zelenko treated over 500 "Covid" patients with hydroxychloroquine + zinc + azitromycine. He also had a 100% recovery rate, with hardly any side effects, and no hospitalizations. As time passed by, Dr. Zelenko helped already 1,000 "Covid" patients recover, usually in a matter of days. He developed a protocol to treat "COVID-19" which became world famous and is saving the lives of tens of thousands of people around the world.

It is called The Zelenko Protocol and consists of administering hydroxychloroquine, combined with zinc and azitromycine.

Hydroxychloroquine is the gun that shoots the bullet (= zinc) and azitromycine is a protective vest.

Ref: https://zelenkoprotocols.co.uk/

There was never any need for the DEADLY "VACCINES"

Dr. Brian Tyson is the owner of 'All Valley Urgent Care' in El Centro, California USA. He has treated over 1,700 corona patients using the **Zelenko Protocol** and saw a 100% recovery rate.

Dr. Stella Immanuel from Texas USA treated over 500 "Covid" patients, with a 100% success rate. Some of them were in their nineties, eighties and seventies. Nobody died! In a broadcast of the **American Frontline Doctors** Dr. Immanuel explains how in Africa this medicine has been used for decades and is even given to new-borns and very elderly, because it's so safe and powerful.

Dr. Immanuel has set up a nationwide TeleMedicine Service USA which you can call, to get prevention and treatment for "COVID-19".

Ref: **https://rehobothmedicalcenter.com/telehealth-service/**

Study from 2005 Proved Anti-viral Effect of Hydroxychloroquine 'HCQ'

The strong anti-viral effect of chloroquine on SARS-CoV had already been proven by an extensive scientific study by the NIH (which is directed by Dr. Anthony Fauci) in 2005. The conclusion of this study was:

'Chloroquine has strong antiviral effects on SARS-CoV infection of primate cells. Chloroquine is effective in preventing the spread of SARS-CoV in cell culture.'

Quercetin as alternative for hydroxychloroquine

A very good alternative to HCQ is a natural supplement called **QUERCETIN**, which does the same thing as HCQ: it helps zinc break through the cell wall and do it's lifesaving job.

Quercetin can be easily purchased in health stores, or you can find it online.

Cure No 2: The Holistic Approach: Hydrogen Peroxide

Dr. David Brownstein, MD developed a second proven, safe and effective cure for "COVID-19" was developed by Dr. David Brownstein from Michigan. Dr. Brownstein has over thirty years of experience in holistic medicine and has been an innovator and pioneer in this field.

Being an experienced holistic practitioner Dr. Brownstein started treating his "Covid" patients with a natural and safe protocol that includes intravenous vitamin C and iodine, nebulized hydrogen peroxide, along with oral administration of vitamins A and D. In an interview with Highwire (which was censored by YouTube) Dr. Brownstein said the following:

'We've treated over a hundred patients and they're all better. No one has been hospitalised or ventilated. We had a 100% success rate with this.

We treated patients who were very old and very sick, and we thought they were dying. But these patients are getting better with these therapies.'

Dr. Joseph Mercola, A world leader in science based education about Natural Health is Doctor Joseph Mercola. This internationally recognized pioneer has been the recipient of numerous awards and honours. In 2009, Dr. Mercola was named the top Ultimate Wellness Game Changer.

Dr. Mercola confirms the efficiency of hydrogen peroxide in defeating respiratory infections and summarizes how it works:

'Hydrogen peroxide sits inside and outside cells of your cells in low levels, ready and waiting to be generated in greater amounts as soon as a pathogen is detected by your immune system.

Nebulizing hydrogen peroxide into your sinuses, throat and lungs is a simple, straightforward way to augment your body's natural expression of hydrogen peroxide to combat infections.

In addition to having direct viricidal effects, iodine improves white blood cell function and thyroid hormone production. This provides a metabolic boost to white blood cells to increase hydrogen peroxide antimicrobial properties which is one way your immune system works to kill pathogens.

Vitamin C also increases hydrogen peroxide production when used at high doses, while vitamin A helps modulate your immune system.

Buy a desktop nebulizer and stock food-grade hydrogen peroxide, Lugol's iodine, and some saline. That way, you have everything you need and can begin treatment at home at the first signs of a respiratory infection.'

In 1920 a study was done by 'The Lancet' to see if intravenous hydrogen peroxide could save the life of dying patients in India, who suffered from an extreme case of broncho-pneumonia of influenzal origin. The result was amazing:

More than 50% of the dying patients - who were considered hopeless by the medical staff - fully recovered.

Cure No 3: Nebulized Budesonide

Dr. Richard Bartlett, MD was asked by Texas USA governor Perry to be part of the Health Disparity Taskforce, which advices the governor on how to establish quality healthcare in all of Texas. Dr. Bartlett was asked year after year again, for seven years, to be on this team. He has also been the health expert for the CBS affiliate in West Texas for 20 years. Furthermore Dr. Bartlett does a weekly update on "COVID-19" on the NewsTalk 550 in West Texas, which he has done since the beginning of this "drama".

Since the pandemic started, Dr. Bartlett successfully treated over 500 COVID-19 patients with a 100% success rate, using a well-known asthma medicine Budesonide.

This treatment is also used in Taiwan, Japan and Iceland, where very few people have died from "Covid-19", in populations of tens of millions of people!

In an interview with 'America can we talk' Dr. Bartlett shares how a lady who was already suffering from two cancers and whose body was weak from the chemo therapies, got "COVID-19" on top of that. She was dying...

The lady was treated with Budesonide and a few days later she worked eight hour shifts again.

Quote: **Prof. Dan Nicolau, University of Oxford**

'...if we keep 60 percent of people out of hospital using budesonide, then, well, that's the kind of thing we throw a barbecue over.'

Other Doctors performing similar excellent work are:

Dr. Jeffrey Barke, MD – 'Covid-19 A Physician's Take on the Exaggerated Fear of the Coronavirus'

Ref: https://www.amazon.com/Covid-19-Physicians-Take-Exaggerated-Coronavirus/dp/0935047948

Professor Peter McCullough, MD, MPH - Speaking at a Senate Committee on Health and Human Services posted: 11th March 2021

Quote: ***'50,000 Research papers about "Covid19" and not one of them told the readership [Doctors] how to treat "Covid19"'***

'I released four slides of a very important research presentation on YouTube and the material went viral. However, YouTube deleted it!'

[For violating their noble sense of deontological ethics!?]

'There was a near total block on any information about treatment of ["Covd19"] ***patients.'***

'[The "Covid19" healthcare and treatment provision] ***was a total failure on every level.'***

[Many social media organisations appear to be instruments of the suppression of important information rather than the liberators or informers thereof.]

'What has gone on is beyond belief!!'

Ref: https://www.youtube.com/watch?v=QAHi3lX3oGM

Dr. Pierre Kory, MD, MPA

Dr. Kory and his team of top medical experts studied the entire medical literature for over nine months and found that Ivermectin proves to be a miracle drug that effectively prevents and treats "COVID-19".

Cure No. 4: Ivermectin

63 peer reviewed studies confirm the effectiveness of Ivermectin in treating "COVID"

Biophysicist Andreas Kalcker used chlorine dioxide to slash the daily death rate of 100 to 0, in Bolivia and was asked to treat the military, police, and politicians in several Latin American nations. His worldwide network 'COMUSAV.com' consists of thousands of physicians, academics, scientists, and lawyers who are promoting this effective treatment.

With several options to successfully treat "COVID-19", why is there still such an outcry for a "vaccine"? **And why is the majority of the population not even aware of the available treatments?** The answer is shocking and shows once more what is going on in our world...

All over the world physicians who were successfully treating "Covid" patients, encountered the unthinkable: they were intimidated and shut down by the government.

America's Frontline Doctors informed the world about the safe and effective cures for "Covid", during their first White Coat Summit in 2020. This broadcast was viewed over twenty million times in a few hours, but then they were shut down - all across the board: Facebook, YouTube, Twitter, and even their own website was taken down by Squarespace.

Front Line COVID-19 Critical Care Alliance (FLCCC)
Another group of medical practioners in the field of cures for "Covid" is the FLCCC as above.

The Cures above are supported/augmented by reports from the FCCC which cover:

Protection Protocol, Early Treatment, Long Covid Treatment, Nutritional Therapeutics, Vitamins and Nutraceuticals during pregnancy.

Founded by a group of leading critical care specialists in March 2020, the Front Line COVID-19 Critical Care Alliance (FLCCC) is dedicated to helping prevent and treat "COVID".

They aim to save lives and improve health by advancing protocols based on the latest science, data, and clinical observations. Their founding physicians are highly published and world-renowned thought leaders, with deep knowledge and expertise to diagnose and treat "COVID"-related symptoms.

To date, the organisation has reached millions of people through its protocols, website, webinars, newsletters, social media, speaking engagements and media appearances. Our protocols are in use by healthcare providers around the world and have helped many thousands of people.

FLCCC is a 501(c)(3) non-profit funded entirely by voluntary donations from individuals and charitable organizations.

FLCCC: A Guide to the Prevention of "COVID-19"

The 'I-PREVENT' protocol must be part of an overall strategy that includes common sense public health actions such as good hand hygiene, avoiding crowded public gatherings, adequate ventilation and other measures. The following protocol can be used for both chronic and post-exposure prevention.

Chronic prevention is especially recommended for healthcare workers, those over 60 years old with comorbidities, people who are morbidly obese, and residents of long-term care facilities. Follow post-exposure prevention if a household member is "COVID"-positive or if you have had prolonged exposure to "COVID" but have not developed symptoms. At the onset of any flu-like symptoms, please refer to the I-CARE Early Treatment Protocol.

About this Protocol

The information in this document is our recommended approach to "COVID-19" based on the best (and most recent) literature. It is provided as guidance to healthcare providers worldwide on the early treatment of "COVID-19". Patients should always consult with their provider before starting any medical treatment. New medications may be added and/or changes made to doses of existing medications as further evidence emerges. Please return to our website at often to be sure you are using the latest version of this protocol.

For more information on nutritional therapeutics and how they can help with "COVID-19", visit our guide to Nutritional Therapeutics. For more information on vitamins and nutraceuticals during pregnancy, visit our guide to Vitamins and Nutraceuticals During Pregnancy.

For additional information on early treatment, the rationale behind these medications, and other optional treatments, see A Guide to Early Treatment of COVID-19. Early treatment is critical and the most important factor in managing this disease.

Chronic Prevention

- **Ivermectin:** 0.2 mg/kg – start treatment with one dose, take second dose 48 hours later, then 1 dose every 7 days (weekly).
  Those at high risk of contracting "COVID-19" can consider dosing twice a week. Due to a possible interaction between quercetin and ivermectin, these drugs should be staggered throughout the day. For COVID treatment, ivermectin is best taken with a meal or just following a meal, for greater absorption.

- **Zinc:** 30-40 mg daily.
  Zinc supplements come in various forms (e.g., zinc sulfate, zinc citrate and zinc gluconate)

- **Melatonin:** Begin with 1 mg and increase as tolerated to 6 mg before bedtime (causes drowsiness).
  Slow- or extended-release formulations preferred.

- **Mouthwash:** 3 times a day.
  Gargle three times a day (do not swallow) with an antiseptic-antimicrobial mouthwash containing chlorhexidine, cetylpyridinium chloride (e.g., Scope™, Act™, Crest™) or povidone-iodine.

- **Steam Inhalation:** once a day.
  Inhaled steam supplemented with antimicrobial essential oils (e.g., Vicks VapoRub™ inhalations) has been demonstrated to have virucidal activity. Antimicrobial essential oils include lavender, thyme, peppermint, cinnamon, eucalyptus and sage.

- **Vitamin D:** dosing varies (see tables below).
  Vitamin D supplementation is likely a highly effective and cheap intervention to lessen the impact of this disease, particularly in vulnerable populations, (i.e., the elderly, obese, people of colour, and those living in northern latitudes).

  The greatest "COVID" protection benefit from Vitamin D supplementation will occur in individuals deficient in Vitamin D. Those individuals should take Vitamin D prophylactically on a longer-term basis. When a person with Vitamin D deficiency develops COVID-19, risks increase for developing complications, and Vitamin D supplementation subsequent to infection will have less of a response.

  Dosing recommendations for Vitamin D supplementation vary widely. The optimal target is over 50 ng/ml; at this level the risk of dying from "COVID-19" is extremely reduced. It may take many months or years to achieve optimal levels in patients who are extremely Vitamin D deficient.

It is therefore important that the optimal regimen for Vitamin D supplementation for the prophylaxis of "COVID-19" is provided promptly, based on baseline Vitamin D levels. If baseline levels are unknown, the needed dose can be calculated from body weight or BMI.

- **Curcumin (turmeric):** 500 mg twice a day.
  Curcumin has low solubility in water and is poorly absorbed by the body; consequently, it is traditionally taken with full fat milk and black pepper, which enhance its absorption.

- **Nigella sativa (black cumin):** 80 mg/kg daily and **Honey** 1g/kg daily.
  Note: thymoquinone (the active ingredient of Nigella sativa) decreases the absorption of cyclosporine and phenytoin. Patients taking these drugs should therefore avoid taking Nigella sativa.

- **Vitamin C:** 500-1000 mg twice a day.

- **Quercetin (or a mixed flavonoid supplement):** 250 mg twice a day.
  Due to a possible interaction between quercetin and ivermectin, these drugs should not be taken simultaneously (i.e., should be staggered at different times of day). As supplemental quercetin has poor solubility and low oral absorption, lecithin-based and nanoparticle formulations are preferred.

- **Probiotics**
  Low levels of Bifidobacterium may predispose a person to COVID-19 and increase disease severity. Likewise, COVID-19 depletes the microbiome of Bifidobacterium, which may then increase the severity and duration of symptoms. Kefir (a fermented milk drink) is high in Bifidobacterium and other probiotics that have demonstrated health benefits. Suggested probiotic supplements include Megasporebiotic (Microbiome labs), TrueBifidoPro (US Enzymes) and yourgutplus+.

  NOTE: Depending on the brand, these products can be very high in sugar, which promotes inflammation. Look for brands without added sugar or fruit jellies and choose products with more than one strain of lactobacillus and bifidobacteria. Try to choose probiotics that are also gluten free, casein free and soy free.

Ref: https://covid19criticalcare.com/treatment-protocols/

CHAPTER 16

HOW TO MINIMISE "COVID19" "VACCINE" ADVERSE EFFECTS

Legal Notice: It is understood that at the time of publication, that not all of the "Covid19" "vaccine" side effects can be fully remedied. It is hoped that this will not be the case with the application of further, future research.

INTRODUCTION

Please note below the civil and criminal prosecutions of some of Big Pharma

Year	Company	Settlement	USA Laws violated
2012	GlaxoSmithKline	\$3 billion (\$1B criminal, \$2B civil)	False Claims Act, FDCA
2009	Pfizer	\$2.3 billion (\$1.189B criminal)	False Claims Act, FDCA
2013	Johnson & Johnson	\$2.2 billion	False Claims Act, FDCA

The Pfizer fine of \$2.3 billion (\$1.189B criminal) was the largest criminal fine in USA History for any offence! Would YOU indemnify a criminal company?

Ref 1: https://en.wikipedia.org/wiki/List_of_largest_pharmaceutical_settlements

Ref 2: **Pfizer Criminality, USA Justice Department:** Url link: https://www.justice.gov/opa/pr/justice-department-announces-largest-health-care-fraud-settlement-its-history

Pfizer Documents Produced by the FDA in Freedom of Information act FOIA Litigation

Ref 1: https://www.icandecide.org/pfizer/

Ref2: https://icandecide.org/article/pfizers-documents-public-health-and-medical-professionals-for-transparency-documents-november-1-2022/

<u>Confidential paper from Pfizer that lists c. 10 pages, 2,291-word count Adverse Side Effects associated with their "COVID" "vaccine"</u>. And Pfizer wanted to keep this horror story private for 75 years!! That act in itself must surely be criminal!

Pfizer Adverse Event Reports Received Through 28-Feb-2021 (pdf) 38-Page Pfizer Report with 10-page Appendix – see below:

Ref: https://sunfellow.com/wp-content/uploads/2022/03/5.3.6-postmarketing-experience.pdf

The **Pfizer ONLY "vaccine",** showing 2,291-word count, 10 pages of Adverse Side Effects from this document above are listed in full in APPENDIX III.

The best way to minimise "Covid19" "vaccine" adverse side effects is to NOT take the "vaccines". It would be illegal for it to be forced upon you. Informed consent is an imperative.

Furthermore, the human body is a very cleverly designed set of interconnected organs and in order for it to strive to perpetuate its existence, which is inherent in all creatures because it is inherent in Natural Law, it has built up over years and years and years of its existence an extraordinary immune system. It may well be wiser to do ALL you can to strengthen your immune system using a balanced healthy diet, ample sensible exercise such as swimming, remove unnecessary stress (i.e., the stupid need to have more material objects and the more expensive, material objects the better than your colleagues, friends, and neighbours so that you can fool yourself into thinking such objects make you superior in some way), go to bed early, get a good night's sleep etc. etc. rather than lay your body on the alter-slab of Big Pharma. BMW cars are not named 1,3,5,7 series for no reason. The pauper starts his slavery buying BMW 1 series with debt money and chains himself to this lifetime of debt slavery as he proceeds up the greasy pole to Nirvana on Earth, the BMW 7 series!

The obvious paradox of Big Pharma is that they cannot be in the business of making sick people well, because if one tablet could cure all diseases then they would be out of business very soon indeed. No, they must be in the business of NOT curing, but CONTAINING the symptoms of disease. In this way, the 'patient-slave' is, for the rest of their lives, under the drug-yoke of the pharmaceutical company and the NHS/insurance company premiums to pay for the privilege of the 'patient-slave' perpetual misery of enslavement.

Health services will never truly work under this capitalist drug-yoke. The solution is simple. As stated above regarding the human immune system together with natural remedies wherever possible.

"Covid19" "vaccines" contain Graphene Oxide in Varying Degrees of Toxicity

Graphene oxide, a substance that is poisonous to humans, has been found in the "Covid19" "vaccines". Graphene oxide interacts, and is activated by, electromagnetic frequencies ("EMF"), specifically the broader range of frequencies found in 5G which can cause even more damage to our health. The symptoms of graphene oxide poisoning, and EMF radiation sickness, are similar to those symptoms described as "Covid". Now that graphene oxide has been identified as a contaminant, there are ways to remove graphene oxide from your body and restore your health.

This is a holistic approach of using several different methods simultaneously for the best effect. Including, specific supplements to degrade the graphene oxide in the body and controlling EMFs in the environment to minimize graphene oxide activation.

This information comes from several sources and is based on scientific studies. Links are referenced below.

Understanding Glutathione

Glutathione is a substance made from the amino acids: glycine, cysteine, and glutamic acid. It is produced naturally by the liver and involved in many processes in the body, including tissue building and repair, making chemicals and proteins needed in the body, and for the immune system. We have a natural glutathione reserve in our bodies. This is what gives us a strong immune system.

When glutathione levels are high in the body, we have no problems and our immune system functions well. But when the amount of graphene oxide in the body exceeds the amount of glutathione, it causes the collapse of the immune system and triggers a cytokine storm. The way that graphene oxide can rapidly grow to exceed glutathione in the body is by electronic excitation. Meaning, EMF's that bombard the graphene to oxidise it, which rapidly triggers the disease.

At the age of 65 years, glutathione levels fall drastically in the body. This can explain why the population most affected by Covid-19 are the elderly. Glutathione levels are also very low in people with pre-existing conditions such as diabetes, obesity, etc. Likewise, glutathione levels are very high in infants, children, and athletes. This can explain why Covid-19 has not affected these people.

Graphene oxide when oxidised or activated by specific EMF frequencies overruns the body's ability to create enough glutathione, which destroys the immune system and causes the illness. In events of illness (such as Covid symptoms and all the "variants") it is necessary to raise glutathione levels in the body in order to cope with the toxin (graphene oxide) that has been introduced or electrically activated.

ICU Intubated Covid Patients Healed Within Hours When Treated with Glutathione And NAC, Example from Ricardo Delgado

"We have seen clinical trials with hundreds of patients who were in the ICU, on a respirator and intubated, practically on the verge of death. With bilateral pneumonias caused by the spread of graphene oxide and subsequent 5G radiation in the lung plaques. Well, this diffuse stain in these patients is symmetrical, which would not happen with a biological agent since it would be rather asymmetrical, as for example when there is a pneumococcal infection, right? Well, in that case a diffuse stain usually appears in one part of the lung, but not in another, not in both symmetrically. So, when treated with glutathione via direct intravenous —or even orally as well— or with N-acetylcysteine (NAC) 600 mg or higher doses, people within hours began to recover their oxygen saturation" – Ricardo Delgado, *La Quinta Colmuna*

N-acetylcysteine ("NAC") is a supplement that causes the body to produce glutathione, it is known as the precursor to glutathione and causes the body to secrete glutathione endogenously, just as it does when you do sports intensely. NAC comes from the amino acid L-cysteine and is used by the body to build antioxidants. Antioxidants are vitamins, minerals, and other nutrients that protect and repair cells from damage. You can get NAC as a supplement or a prescription drug.

Zinc in combination with NAC are essential antioxidants used to degrade graphene oxide. Ricardo Delgado states that with these two antioxidants he has personally helped people affected by magnetism after inoculation. This is in people with two doses of Pfizer who have become magnetic and after these supplements they no longer have this symptom.

Other supplements that can be taken to assist in the removal of graphene oxide are:

- Astaxanthin
- Melatonin
- Milk Thistle
- Quercetin
- Vitamin C
- Vitamin D3

Ref: https://www.holistichealthonline.info/product/graphene-removal/

Ref: https://expose-news.com/2022/10/30/guide-how-to-remove-graphene-from-body/

"Covid19" "vaccines" contain other Harmful Elements in Varying Degrees of Toxicity

Josep Pàmies discusses these other Harmful Elements and how one might deal with them in the interview below:

***Josep Pàmies* 'How to Detoxify the Body With Natural Infusions'**

Interviewer:

'As you rightly said, those people that, even though, may have had the information at their fingertips, have taken a dose ["Covid19" "vaccination"] *because they felt pressed and gave in. And we still must try to make sure that, at least, they don't take the second dose. And if they've taken it, don't go take a third, a fourth, a fifth... Try to get out of that cycle. What's your recommendation for those people?'*

Josep Pàmies:

'We don't know if all the crap* [from "Covid19" "vaccines"] *will come out with what we recommend, but a lot of it will. That's to say, the liver and kidney have to be in perfect condition. If they are not, you have to start taking hepatic and renal herbs.

Hepatic in the morning and renal in the evening or afternoon.

Which ones are hepatic? ***Dandelion, milk thistle, desmodium. Those are basic plants for the liver.***

For the kidney, dandelion can be taken as well, horsetail grass, and nettle.

Those are plants that will improve the functioning of the kidney and liver, which are the filters of our blood.'

'When there are heavy metals, which there will be, we must add, for example, Tulsi, which is a sacred plant from India. It's called ***Tulsi (Ocimum Sanctum)****. Or you can use* ***Houttuynia cordata****.*

Those are two potent plants that help in detoxifying poisons, heavy metals, and are also helpful for radioactivity.

Be careful, eh? ***We don't know what shit they have put in the "vaccines"****.*

Houttuynia cordata, for example, is the plant that was used in Hiroshima and Nagasaki to save a lot of people*. I have met —through a Catalan friend who is in Japan sponsored by a Japanese family— a man of about 100 years old who lived in that house.*

He was affected by radiation in Hiroshima. He was the only one who survived in his family because he was the only one treated with these infusions. *They had few plants.*

When this girl (my friend) asked to do an investigation in Japan, together with public organizations here in Spain and Japan, she found quite a long list of survivors of Hiroshima and Nagasaki.

All of them had used that plant, Houttuynia cordata.

*When we study that plant... If you look up '****Houttuynia cordata****' in the PubMed medical search engine, you'll learn that it's quite amazing for treating SARS-CoV-2 (or 1 or whatever), for detoxifying from snake venom of any kind.'*

'And another substance that we have to take to finish cleaning our bodies, is ***activated charcoal****.*

There are protocols on how to take activated charcoal. It's totally harmless. In the immense porosity that this charcoal has inside the body, all the filth that may come from "vaccines" or from other food sources or... Who knows! Even meds we have taken are lodged. And the charcoal cleanses the organism.'

'What's done in hospitals when there's an intoxication is to treat patients with activated charcoal. We can do it at home. They sell it. You have to become familiar with it.'

'Another effective treatment is zeolite. ***Zeolite is another mineral that also adsorbs crap that we may have in the body.*** *And it helps us excrete it through faeces or urine.'*

'So, we have zeolite, activated charcoal, and then the plants I have recently mentioned to remove the heavy metals in our bodies (Tulsi and Houttuynia cordata).'

'Basically, they are plants to improve the functioning of the kidney, the liver, as I have already told you before. That's the basics.'

By ***Josep Pàmies*** **'How to Detoxify the Body with Natural Infusions'**

Ref: https://www.orwell.city/2021/08/josep-pamies.html

Front Line COVID-19 Critical Care Alliance (FLCCC)

As described in the previous chapter the FLCCC group assist in treatments for **"Covid19"**.

They also offer treatments for illness after one has been "vaccinated" against "Covid19"

Ref: https://covid19criticalcare.com/ **Front Line COVID-19 Critical Care Alliance (FLCCC)**

FLCCC POST-VACCINE TREATMENT PROTOCOL

Management of Post-Vaccine Syndrome

Major public health authorities do not recognize post-COVID-vaccine injuries no specific ICD classification code exists for this disease. However, while no official definition exists, a temporal correlation between receiving a COVID-19 vaccine and the beginning or worsening of a patient's clinical manifestations is sufficient to diagnose a COVID-19 vaccine-induced injury, when symptoms are otherwise unexplained by concurrent causes.

Since there are no published reports detailing how to manage vaccine-injured patients, our treatment approach is based on the postulated pathogenetic mechanism, clinical observation, and patient anecdotes. Treatment must be individualized according to each patient's presenting symptoms and disease syndromes. Chances are, not all patients will respond equally to the same intervention; a particular intervention may be lifesaving for one patient and completely ineffective for another.

Early treatment is essential; the response to treatment will most likely be attenuated when treatment is delayed.

About this Protocol

This document is primarily intended to assist healthcare professionals in providing appropriate medical care for vaccine-injured patients. Patients should always consult a trusted healthcare provider before embarking on any new treatment.

First Line Therapies

- **Intermittent daily fasting** or periodic daily fasts.
  Fasting stimulates the clearing of damaged cells (autophagy), damaged mitochondria (mitophagy), and misfolded and foreign proteins. Fasting is contraindicated in patients younger than 18 (impairs growth), malnourished patients (BMI < 20 kg/m2), and during pregnancy and breastfeeding. Patients with diabetes, gout, or serious underlying medical conditions should consult their primary care provider before beginning fasting, as changes in medications may be required and these patients require close monitoring. See page 4 for quick tips on fasting. For more detailed information see 'An Approach to the Management of Post-Vaccine Syndrome'.

- **Ivermectin:** 0.2-0.3 mg/kg/day
  Ivermectin, which has potent anti-inflammatory properties, binds to the spike protein and aids in its elimination. It is likely that ivermectin and intermittent fasting act synergistically to rid the body of spike protein. Ivermectin is best taken with or just following a meal for greater absorption. A trial of ivermectin should be included in the first-line treatment approach. The duration of treatment is determined by the clinical response. In patients with a suboptimal response, a trial of a higher dose (0.6mg/kg day) can be considered. If no improvement is noted after 4-6 weeks, the drug should be stopped. Due to the possible drug interaction between quercetin and ivermectin, these drugs should not be taken simultaneously (i.e., should be staggered morning and night). The safety of ivermectin in pregnancy is uncertain, therefore this drug should be avoided in the first trimester of pregnancy.

- **Moderating physical activity:**
  Patients with long COVID and post-vaccine symptoms frequently suffer from severe post-exertional fatigue and/or worsening of symptoms with exercise. Aerobic exercise is reported to be one of the worst therapeutic interventions for these patients. We recommend moderating activity to tolerable levels that do not worsen symptoms, keeping the patient's heart rate under 110 BPM. Furthermore, patients need to identify the activity level beyond which their symptoms worsen, and then aim to stay below that level of activity. Stretching and low-level resistance exercises are preferred over aerobic exercises.

- **Low Dose Naltrexone (LDN)**:
  LDN has been demonstrated to have anti-inflammatory, analgesic, and neuromodulating properties. Begin with 1 mg/day and increase to 4.5 mg/day, as required. May take 2 to 3 months to see full effect.

- **Resveratrol**
  This plant phytochemical (flavonoid) has remarkable biological properties and activates autophagy. A bio-enhanced formulation containing trans-resveratrol from Japanese Knotweed Root appears to have improved bioavailability. Quercetin acts synergistically and increases the bioavailability of resveratrol. Pterostilbene is another plant flavonoid similar to resveratrol, but with greater absorption and cellular uptake. A "high quality" combination supplement with resveratrol, quercetin, and pterostilbene is ideal. Resveratrol in a dose of 500 mg twice daily is suggested for acutely symptomatic patients. In recovered patients and those on preventative/maintenance therapy, a daily dose of 400-500 mg should suffice. The safety of these phytochemicals has not been determined in pregnancy and they should therefore be avoided. Due to the possible drug interaction between quercetin and ivermectin these drugs should not be taken simultaneously (i.e., should be staggered morning and night). For more detailed information see 'An Approach to the Management of Post-Vaccine Syndrome'.

- **Melatonin:** 2–6 mg slow release/extended release prior to bedtime.
  Melatonin has anti-inflammatory and antioxidant properties and is a powerful regulator of mitochondrial function. The dose should be started at 750 mcg (μg) to 1 mg at night and increased as tolerated. Patients who are slow metabolizers may have very unpleasant and vivid dreams with higher doses.

- **Aspirin:** 81 mg/day.

- **Probiotics/prebiotics**
  Patients with post-vaccine syndrome classically have severe dysbiosis with loss of Bifidobacterium. A no-sugar-added, Greek yogurt with both pre- and probiotics is recommended. Suggested probiotics include Megasporebiotic (Microbiome labs), TrueBifidoPro (US Enzymes) and yourgutplus+. Depending on the brand, some pro/prebiotic products can be very high in sugar, which promotes inflammation, so read labels carefully.

- **Sunlight and Photobiomodulation (PBM)**
  PBM is also referred to as low-level light therapy, red light therapy, and near-infrared light therapy. Of all the wavelengths of sunlight, near-infrared radiation (NIR-A) has the deepest penetration into tissues. NIR-A in the range of 1000 to 1500 nm is optimal for heating tissues. For more detailed information see 'An Approach to the Management of Post-Vaccine Syndrome'.

Further details are available on the URL link below.

Ref: https://covid19criticalcare.com/treatment-protocols/i-recover/

FLCCC Disclaimer:

FLCCC protocols are solely for educational purposes regarding potentially beneficial therapies for COVID-19. Never disregard professional medical advice because of something you have read on our website and releases. This protocol is not intended to be a substitute for professional medical advice, diagnosis, or treatment with regard to any patient. Treatment for an individual patient should rely on the judgement of a physician or other qualified health provider. Always seek their advice with any questions you may have regarding your health or medical condition. Please note FLCCC full disclaimer at: www.flccc.net/disclaimer

[**LEGAL AND MEDICAL NOTE**: It may be wise to ensure that all medical advice that a reader may receive is independent morally, technically, and financially from any bias, is provided by a competent professional in the appropriate technical field, and that there is no conlfict of interest regarding the situation appertaining to the advice provider.]

Ref: https://covid19criticalcare.com/treatment-protocols/ for all FACT SHEETS:

FACT SHEET 2: Diagnostic Lab Tests for Evaluation of Injury Following COVID Shots

This list is provided as an educational resource for our readers and supporters. This is not an exhaustive list, but it reflects the integrated evaluation I have done for my medical patients for many years, with added inflammatory and other markers that I have found particularly important to evaluate my patients who have developed new medical conditions after the experimental COVID shots.

Inflammation, micro-blood clotting, and susceptibility to atypical viral and bacterial infections are common after the COVID shots, so I have recommended to my patients that we check these (and other) markers to assess risk and decide treatment. I have organized them into the categories related to types of medical problems I am seeing in my independent medical practice. I have provided my list to help people know that there ARE tests you can request to help answer your questions and decide what treatments may help relieve your symptoms.

Each of you reading this will need to discuss with your own health professionals what is appropriate for you based on medical evaluation of your particular symptoms. Join our discussion group on Vaccine Injury on our Clout Hub channel: @TruthForHealth

~Elizabeth Lee Vliet, MD, President and CEO Truth for Health Foundation

METABOLIC TESTS:

Comprehensive Metabolic Profile
Glycosylated hemoglobin
CBC with differential
Vitamin B6 and B1
Magnesium (serum and RBC)
Cholesterol profile
Fasting insulin
Vitamin B12, Folate
25-OH Vitamin D
Zinc

ENDOCRINE TESTS - Draw in AM prior to any meds to assess damage to endocrine system

FSH, LH, Estradiol, Progesterone, Testosterone (free and total), DHEA-S, DHEA
TSH (hs), Free T3 and Free T4, Anti-microsomal, Anti-thyroglobulin AB
8 AM Cortisol, total and free, Prolactin, Parathyroid Hormone, Amylase, Lipase
PSA, CA125, CA 19-9, CEA, CA 15-9

INFLAMMATORY MARKERS and SPECIALTY TESTS:

CRP-hs Fibrinogen D-Dimer Troponin-1
Ferritin Cytokine Panel IL-6, IL-10 Myeloperoxidase (MPO)
24-hour urine for measure of: catecholamines, metanephrines, VMA

To assess new infections:
SARS-CoV-2 spike protein antibodies
SARS-CoV-2 Nucleocapsid Antibodies
Mycoplasma pneumoniae, EBV titers, CMV titers, RSV titers
HIV and other viral titers as indicated by presenting symptoms.

FACT SHEET 2 Addition: Specialty Diagnostic Imaging Tests for Evaluation of Injury Following COVID Shots:

This list is provided as an educational resource for our readers and supporters. This is not an exhaustive list, but it reflects the specialty imaging studies I have researched in consultation with radiology experts. I have found these tests critically important to evaluate my medical patients with new onset medical problems after the experimental COVID shots and suspected of being related to vaccine-induced inflammation and abnormal blood clotting. There are other specialty imaging studies that can be ordered based on each patient's cluster of symptoms and signs. Readers will need to discuss with their health professionals what is appropriate based on individual medical evaluation.

~Elizabeth Lee Vliet, MD, President and CEO Truth for Health Foundation

- CT Temporal Bone, high-resolution
  Clinical symptoms: dizziness, vertigo, impaired balance, suspected injury to ossicles
  Need detailed assessment of whether ossicles are intact. With contrast at discretion of neuroradiologist

- 3 Tesla MRI brain, with and without contrast, WITH Internal Auditory Canal (IAC) Protocol and attention to posterior fossa structures
  Clinical Symptoms: dizziness, vertigo, impaired balance, impaired cognition, abnormal sensation (numbness, tingling), other: ______________

- Cardiac MRI for morphology and function, with late-phase gadolinium enhancement to assess for myocarditis, pericarditis
  Clinical symptoms: chest pain, palpitations, arrythmias

- CT Angiogram of Lung with arterial and venous phases to evaluate for peripheral microthrombi and/or larger pulmonary emboli
  Clinical symptoms: shortness of breath, dyspnea on exertion

Other specialty studies can be ordered to assess gastrointestinal pain syndromes, suspected abdominal and/or pelvic blood clots, ovarian or testicular pain syndromes following the experimental COVID shots.

Ref: https://www.truthforhealth.org/wp-content/uploads/2022/05/2022-VaccineInjuryTreatmentGuide_4-29-22-FINAL.pdf

Also Generic Ref: https://www.truthforhealth.org/

FACT SHEET 3: Prevention and Treatment Options – Nutraceuticals, Foods, Supplements

This FACT SHEET is designed to be a rapid action plan checklist of steps you can take on your own, without a physician's prescription, to create your Health Action Plan. For more details on the options in our master list, please refer to the references section, and the more detailed Fact Sheets on these areas we are adding to our resources regularly. This master list gives you items to create your shopping list to start adding to your home prevention and treatment kit.

FIVE MAIN Goals for both prevention and treatment of COVID vaccine-induced injury (these also apply to COVID illness, and to radiation-induce illness):

- REDUCE SYSTEMIC INFLAMMATION
- REDUCE RISK OF BLOOD CLOTS
- BOOST IMMUNE RESPONSE
- IMPROVE CELLULAR OXYGENATION
- NEUROPROTECTION

I. **REDUCE SYSTEMIC INFLAMMATION**

A. **<u>Supplement and Nutraceutical Options</u>**

- Vitamin D3 2000-4000 IU daily *unless deficient and doses will need to be increased*
- Vitamin C 1000-2000 mg twice a day up to three times a day
- Vitamin E
- Fish Oils
- Turmeric
- Resveratrol
- Monolaurin
- Glucosamine
- Blackseed extract (N. Sativa)
- Chondroitin sulfate - body needs this to build and fix DNA damage
- Green tea (EGCG) and green tea extract 500 mg/day
- Quercetin 500 mg 2-3 times a day
- Glutathione, and/or N-acetyl cysteine (NAC) 600 mg - 1200 mg daily + Glycine 500mg
- Resveratrol 500 mg
- Beta carotene (take with fat to improve absorption)
- Curcumin 500 mg with black pepper (piperine)
- Ginger <2 grams/day ~1600 mg
- Bromelain 500 mg
- Glycine
- Sulfur (found in MSM)
- Melatonin
- Proper balance of Omega 3 Fatty acids (FA) and Omega 6 FA
- Spirulina <8 grams
- Fiber with fructooligosaccharides (FOS)
- Whole food-source multivitamin such a Balance of Nature.
- Probiotics – but avoid ones that are solely Lactobacillus family as over time they alter GI pH in negative direction. Consider a mixed probiotics

that has several different organisms, such as SugarShift, available at www.BiotiQuest.com

B. ANTI-INFLAMMARY FOODS as Medicine - Dietary Approaches:

- **Increase water intake.** Adequate hydration is critical to your health and normal body function. Water is a natural diuretic, and detoxifier, and helps maintain blood volume for circulating nutrients and oxygenation, removal of wastes. You are adequately hydrated if your urine is the color of pale straw. Darker yellow urine means inadequate water intake. Colorless urine means too much water intake and leads to dilutional low sodium and other electrolyte imbalances.
- **Eat a whole food plant-based** diet, limiting processed foods, emphasizing "clean" foods, lean, nonfarm raised protein sources predominantly from bean, legumes, raw nuts and seeds and fish.
- **Increase whole grains** such as barley, rye, oats and lentils, and non-gluten grains
- **Increase cruciferous vegetables,** such as broccoli, Brussel sprouts, cabbage, kale, cauliflower. These are rich in folate, vit C, E and K, and fiber. They also contain glucosinolates that protect cells from DNA damage, inactivate carcinogens, and have anti-bacterial and anti-viral properties.
- **Increase intake of fresh fruits and berries** including apples, bananas, grapefruit, cherries, strawberries, blackberries, and raspberries
- **Eat more in the ALLIUM family of vegetables**: garlic, onions, leeks, chives, scallions, and shallots. These are antioxidants, with anti-viral and anti-bacterial properties. They boost the immune system and can help reduce the risks of blood clotting.
- **Season foods with anti-inflammatory spices**: turmeric, ginger, cinnamon, fennel, fenugreek, coriander, clove allspice, mustard nutmeg, black pepper, garlic and onion powder, cumin, no salt spice blends
- **Use healthy fats**: olive oil and avocado oil in moderation. Eliminate seed oils and polyunsaturated fats from your diet, including vegetable oils
- **Eliminate artificial additives**: sweeteners, flavorings, MSG, dyes, preservatives, sodium and added sugars. These ALL add an inflammatory load to the body.

II REDUCE RISK OF BLOOD CLOTS

A. **Supplement and Nutraceutical Options**

- Vitamins B, C, and E
- Fish oils (Do not take with anti-clotting drugs)
- Co-Q-10
- Ginkgo biloba
- Bromelain
- Probiotics – Avoid ones that are solely Lactobacillus family as over time they alter GI pH in negative direction. Consider a mixed probiotics that has several different organisms, such as SugarShift, available at www.BiotiQuest.com

B. **ANTI-COAGULANT FOODS as Medicine - Dietary Approaches:**

- **Whole grains**: Oats slow cooked or oat groats, whole wheat or wheat berries, rye, barley, brown rice, and quinoa
- **Fresh fruits** including apples, cherries, prunes, pears, citrus
- **Raw nuts**: almonds, pistachios, cashews, walnuts, peanuts
- **Seasonings and Alliums** including garlic, turmeric, cinnamon, cayenne pepper
- **Legumes**, beans, and lentils
- **sunflower** seeds
- **lean proteins** such as skinless white chicken, white-fleshed fish, Greek yogurt, low fat cottage cheese
- **Extra virgin olive oil**
- **Red Wine**

III. BOOST IMMUNE SYSTEM

A. **Supplement and Nutraceutical Supports**:

- **Vitamin D3** 2000-4000 IU daily, unless deficient and doses will need to be increased
- **Vitamin C** 1000-2000 mg twice a day up to three times a day
- **Vitamin B12 and B9**
- **Zinc**
- **Resveratrol**
- **Cocoa Extract**
- **Elderberry Extract**
- **Luteolin**
- **Monolaurin**
- **Melatonin**
- **Ginkgo biloba**
- **Quercetin**
- **N-acetyl cysteine** (NAC) plus glycine
- **Curcumin**
- **Probiotics** – but avoid ones that are solely Lactobacillus family as over time they alter GI pH in negative direction. Consider a mixed probiotics that has several different organisms, such as SugarShift, available at www.BiotiQuest.com

B. **IMMUNE-BOOSTING FOODS as Medicine - Dietary Approaches**:

- **Kefir** (fermented milk, excellent source of healthy bacteria to improve gut microbiome). Avoid commercial products high in sugars. Easy to make your own at home, with "starter" available in health food stores, on-line vitamin, and nutritional supplement sources.
- **Yogurt**, without added sugars, and with live healthy bacteria cultures. Greek-style yogurt has both live cultures and higher protein content.
- **Fresh fruits and vegetables** including citrus fruits, apples. kiwi, bananas, berries, tomatoes, leafy and dark green vegetables, Brussel sprouts, cabbage, radishes, arugula, cauliflower, and bell peppers

- **black currants** and black currant tea
- **Whole grains**: Oats slow cooked or oat groats, whole wheat or wheat berries, rye, barley, brown rice, and quinoa
- **Raw nuts**: almonds, pistachios, cashews, walnuts, peanuts
- **Seeds**: raw sunflower, sesame, hemp, pumpkin, chia
- **Spices**: ginger, turmeric, rosemary, fenugreek, clove, cinnamon, nutmeg, black pepper, cumin, fennel
- **Legumes**, beans, and lentils
- **Mushrooms**, and/or immune-boost Mushroom Complex powder (Lion's Mane, Turkey Tail, Reishi, Maitake, Chaga etc.)
- **Green tea** and anise tea
- **Allium family of vegetables**: onions and garlic, chives, scallions
- **Wild caught seafood and salmon**
- **Dark chocolate**
- **Organic extra virgin olive oil** (cold first pressed)
- **Bone broth**
- **Raw local honey**

IV. IMPROVE CELLULAR OXYGENATION

The goal is to suppress and repair the chain reaction triggered by overproduction of oxygen free radicals or reactive stress species (ROS) and optimize the body's antioxidant defense mechanisms.

A. **<u>Supplement and Nutraceutical Supports:</u>**

- **N-acetyl cysteine** (NAC)
- **Glutathione**
- **Vitamin E**
- **Black seed oil** (N. Sativa seeds, preferably Egyptian). Rich in thymoquinone: eliminates superoxides, is neuroprotective, antioxidant, anti-inflammatory, anti-bacterial, anti-viral

B. **ANTIOXIDANT FOODS as Medicine - Dietary Approaches**:

- **Fresh fruits and green leafy vegetables** including grapes, citrus, pomegranate, spinach and kale
- **Berries**
- **Seasonings and Spices** including turmeric, ginger, cinnamon, and Cayenne pepper
- **ALLIUM family of vegetables**: garlic, onions, leeks, and beetroot
- **Fatty fish** including salmon, trout, and herring
- **Nuts**
- **Chocolate**

V. NEUROPROTECTION

A. <u>Supplement and Nutraceutical Supports</u>:

- **Alpha Lipoic Acid**
- **Grapeseed Extract**

- **Coenzyme Q10** (CoQ10)
- **Sulforaphane**
- **Selenium**
- **N-acetylcysteine** (NAC)
- **Carotenoids**: lycopene, lutein, astaxanthin and zeaxanthin or a mixed carotenoid
- **Vit A, C and E**
- **Resveratrol**
- **Ashwagandha**
- **Sulfur**
- **Zinc**
- **EGCG**
- **Curcumin**
- **Ginkgo biloba L.**
- **Turmeric/ curcumin**

B. **NEUROPROTECTIVE FOODS as Medicine - Dietary Approaches**:

- **Whole Grains**: brown rice, barley, oatmeal, whole-grain breads and pasta
- **Dairy:** milk, yogurt, natural cheese (avoid non-processed cheese products)
- **Fresh vegetables** like asparagus, broccoli, and kale and other leafy greens vegetables
- **Seasonings:** ginger garlic turmeric cassia cinnamon cayenne pepper,
- **Oils:** grape seed extract olive oil
- **Seafood**: tuna, mackerel, salmon, herring, and sardines
- **Nuts and Seeds**: sunflower seeds, almonds, peanuts, raw Brazil nuts, and hazelnuts
- **Dark orange fruits**, apples, grapes, and pineapple
- **Eggs**
- **Avocado**
- **Dark Chocolate**
- **Red wine**
- **Tomatoes**
- **Green tea**
- **Ginseng**
- **Rosemary**
- **Garlic**

VI. CLEAN UP YOUR ENVIRONMENT

A. **Food and Lifestyle**

- **Reduce Alcohol**
- **For the duration of symptoms STOP intake of all inflammatory animal products** including all meats and dairy except grass fed, poultry, and eggs
- **Limit added sugars** including artificial sweeteners
- **Choose whole foods** and **homemade foods** over processed convenience foods or restaurants

- **No smoking**
- **Increase daily physical activity**
- **Turn off negative news**
- **Reduce time on social media**
- **Scripture and Prayer daily**
- **Laughter and play** – find ways to create more "laughter medicine" in your day
- **Practice yoga, Tai Chi, Qi Gong, breathing exercises** to improve relaxation, reduce stress, improve oxygenation, boost immune function
- **Improve your social support** – increase relaxing, fun times with family and friends to reduce stress and improve your well-being

B. **Physical Environment**
   - **INCREASE time outdoors in the sunshine** – walking, gardening, relaxing outside
   - **Reduce 4G/5G exposure** – keep phones out of bedroom, turn off WiFi in home at night, etc.
   - **Reduce your use of synthetic chemicals** and synthetic fragranced products in the home clean with simple vinegar, bleach, alcohol our grandmothers used without all the extra chemicals that increase inflammation and add to vaccine injury

VII. Health and Resilience

- **Resilience** is the capacity to withstand adversity, bounce back, and recover from difficult life events and grow despite life's downturns and setbacks.
- **Resilience** allows us to live fully in this world: mind, body, and spirit, as well as in relationships and in our connections with the environment around us.
- **Our capacity** for resilience, which encompasses all aspects of health, is also an innate gift from our Creator to every man, woman and child. Investing into our relationship with God through His Son, Jesus Christ allows us to tap into the gift of resilience He has given to each of us. God has made this world with many tools and resources for our health and wellbeing. Some of these tools and resources are more commonly known, while others we must use our minds and dig deeper to fully understand and develop new skills for this world.
- **5 Days to Spiritual Vaccination**: Become Immune to Future Worries, Past Wounds, and FindPeace Amidst Trials through Christ and the Christian Mystic Tradition. This is a wonderful, inspiring guide to overcoming the fear and panic we have experienced in the years of the pandemic. https://interiorlife.app/tfh-spiritual-vaccination/
- **Resilience** also means studying the ways that "PsyOps" and psychological tools are used to influence your thoughts, feelings, and decision-making. Check out the Powerpoint presentations on our website under Mind Strategies in the Health and Resilience section. The one by neuroscientist, Dr. Stephen Sammut, is particularly good and enlightening: Neurobiological Basis of Crowd Behavior.

- **Learn more about way**s to achieve resilience for mind, body and spirit health and well-being in our "Health and Resilience" Program at the link below: https://www.truthforhealth.org/resilience/

UNDERSTAND THESE KEY POINTS ABOUT THE "COVID" SHOTS:

- **The experimental COVID shots are not traditional vaccines**. They fall in the FDA regulatory category of gene-therapy agents. The mRNA and DNA are carried into our cells and alter our body's DNA to trigger production of the synthetic spike proteins and disrupt our normal immune system responses.
- **This new technology, never used in vaccines before**, triggers the body to make uncontrolled amounts of the spike proteins that led to unique reactions in the body not seen with traditional vaccines. These three reactions are primarily caused by the synthetic spike protein and by the lipid nanoparticle coating used to carry the mRNA or DNA into the body's cells to alter our own DNA.
    - **An exaggerated inflammatory response**, causing damage to critical organs. In its most serious form, this is called cytokine storm.
    - **An exaggerated blood-clotting response**, leading to multiple blood clots (thrombi) in the lungs, brain, kidneys, intestines and other critical organs. These blood clots can occur in both veins and arteries, which is unusual and potentially life-threatening if not treated rapidly.
    - **Vaccine-induced Acquired Immune Deficiency Syndrome** (VI-AIDS). This means you are more susceptible to all kinds of illness outbreaks - viral, bacterial and fungal, as well as new cancers and recurrence of existing cancers.

Ref: https://www.truthforhealth.org/wp-content/uploads/2022/05/2022-VaccineInjuryTreatmentGuide_4-29-22-FINAL.pdf

[**NOTE:** The above is presented verbatim from the 'Truth For Health Foundation' website given as above, with all appropriate respect for the Religous views expressed concerning God and Jesus Christ.

Theology, Religiosity, Ontology, and Metaphysics, are not subjects covered in this particular essay. These will be dealt with in later works by the Editor of this book.

However, those persons of different faith: Islam, Sufism, Zoroastrianism, Mysticism, Judaism, Buddhism, Hinduism, Sikhism, Cheondoism, Mazdakism, Builders of the Adytum, Asatruism, Eckankarism, Jainism, Aladuraism, CaoDaism, Unification Church, Falun Gong, Lao Tzuism, Confucianism etc. etc. et al are not in any way precluded from the views herein expressed. There can surely, only be **One First Cause**, there may be a few second-tier assistants perhaps, (in the human frame, rather like Michelangelo having assistants to help him paint the Sistine Chapel), but there can be, by the very definition and term, only one First Cause since the Cause is First! The Meaning of Life will be presented in future writings by this Editor. It is not as complicated as people have previously thought.]

CHAPTER 17

HOW TO RETRIEVE YOUR LOSS OF INCOME FROM LOCKDOWN MANDATES & "COVID19" "VACCINES"

Covid Inquiry 2.0 by Senator Malcolm Roberts, Australia - 16th August 2022

Referring to those responsible for the "SarCov2" "Covid19" "pandemic" lies:

'We will hound you down!'

'*It has become clear, the people of this country* [Australia] *and globally have been steamrollered. It is also clear that it has been coordinated globally. It is also clear that it has been integrated not just over 6 months, not just over 2 ½ years, but it has been planned over decades. The changes to legislation in this country were done so that they could control doctors and the people.*

People are awakening and its thanks to Dr Altman and all the presenters here today. ***We know that this*** **["SarCov2" "Covid19" "pandemic"] IS ALL BULLSHIT and we've been HAD.**

But we are going to hound you down. – you people who are guilty. ***We will hound you down and hold you accountable and we will expose you globally, so that the people of Australia look forward to the future, because I love my kids and I'm looking forward to my grandkids.***

We are going to save this country. Thank you.*'*

Ref 1: https://twitter.com/EleonoreNemethM/status/1560878573925404672 20th Aug. 2022

Ref 2: https://rumble.com/v1g95tl-covid-inquiry-2.0.html 16th August 2022

Anyone can be misled, particularly when the persons doing the misleading are very powerful, rich, influential, psychopathic, megalomaniacs bent on total global control.

Anyone can be misled, particularly when the global mass media is in the fearsome grip of the hands of these psychopaths who will not stop at Mass Murder and Genocide to achieve their ends.

Note: "Mass Murder" "Genocide" "psychopaths" "megalomaniacs" are all quotes by Dr Reiner Fuellmich upon consultations with qualified psychologists/psychiatrists via: the strongly recommend video evidence provided, with particular attention to the overview details of this horror, provided in the interview below, (see Ref Url link below), between

Dr Reiner Fuellmich, Attorney and a member of his staff, and Tod Callender US Lawyer, Disabled Rights Advocate, ex-Military – Department of Defence, USA. Mr Callender is currently carrying out lawsuits against the US Government. He raises these and many other very important legal points, supported by his scientific advisers:

1. All those persons "vaccinated" with Pfizer, Moderna etc. have contracted "vaccine"-induced Acquired Immune Deficiency Order 'AIDS'.
2. One injection causes 30% of one's natural immunity to be destroyed.
3. Three injections cause ALL natural immunity to be destroyed. [Tantamount to Murder, and on the global scale of execution, Genocide!]
4. US Insurance companies are expecting circa 5,000% increase in death claims for 2022 – [because of "Covid19" "vaccinations". Similar is anticipated for UK.]
5. US hospitals have already murdered 1M patients. [Similar, proportional numbers are anticipated for UK]. Murder is a three-stage process using "Covid19" "vaccinations".
6. The mRNA "vaccines" – Pfizer, Moderna etc. cause a spike protein at a molecular level within the recipient's body resulting in a form of legal 'transhumanism' whereby the recipient, under current legislation, becomes the lawful property of the person/company that holds the patent on the "vaccine".

Refer to the Dr Reiner Fuellmich, Tod Callender Interview entitled:

'GLOBAL EMERGENCY GENOCIDE EXTINCTION OF MANKIND UNDER WAY'

Ref: Url link: https://www.bitchute.com/video/oRCyqTAEY05o/

Anyone can be misled, particularly when these Evil people have tried this trick before but failed i.e., Swine Flu. They will do anything to not fail a second time.

Anyone can be misled, when the organisations that front this evil are as global, authoritative, powerful, and as well-known as 'Bill and Melinda Gates Foundation', World Health Organisation WHO, World Economic Forum WEF, United Nations UN, The World Bank etc. etc.

Anyone can be misled, if they are told a pack of lies by the "science", or rather the so-called "scientists".

Anyone can be misled, if a complex, multi-faceted, time-dependent matter is reduced to sub-cretinous slogans of perhaps an absolute maximum of two syllables in packs of three. It has been shown that humans have difficulty with trite slogans if the number is not three. One is not enough, two is not enough, four is too many to remember but three has enough cache and amenity to silly little consonantal alliterations (that even Wordsworth would baulk at) that can be readily pummelled into already overworked and tired minds. For example:

'STAY ALERT' 'CONTROL THE VIRUS' 'SAVE LIVES'

This NHS 'genius' stroke of total illiteracy is so appallingly stupid, no wonder the NHS and Baroness Dildo Harding, I believe, wasted £37Bn of taxpayers' hard-earned revenue with their completely useless 'Track and Trace' scheme that anyone in the private sector who failed so miserably with such a scheme, would be completely unemployable for the remainder of this life and possibly the afterlife as well!!

'STAY ALERT'

Don't these blockheads not even know that the typical diameter of a "Covid19" particle is no greater than c. 160Nm? A Nm is 10^{*-9}!! This size relativity may be explained by the metaphor of a marble resting on the North Pole! A marble versus The Earth! Now where did I put my Electron Microscope? I think I left it in the bathroom behind the toothpaste!

'CONTROL THE VIRUS'

Furthermore, how are writers, plumbers, shop keepers, barristers, Law Lords, The Crown, members of The Royal Opera House, premier footballers, David Beckham, funeral directors, prison inmates, Prince Andrew etc. etc. meant to 'Control the Virus'?? I met a man on the Clapham Omnibus back in the days, he was running up and down the bus with a fly-swat – he said he was controlling the virus!

The mind boggles!!

By the time this little 'dialectic' of nonsense arrives at its transcendental, most erudite, philosophical apogee **'SAVE LIVES',** it has well and truly given up the ghost! Why does a person with an IQ of 170/174 (SD 16) top 99.9996599% of the global population have to put up with the nonsense of these idiots? Why are they in Parliament? What use are they? I would not put any of them in charge of an NCP fully computer-controlled Car Park. These people and their nonsense are insulting an intellect of which they know not, nor never will.

We digress.

I could continue this '**Anyone can be misled'** concept for many more pages but it would be pointless to bore the reader.

The point being made is not to reproach yourself, if you regret previous decisions regarding "Covid19" and "vaccines".

Now that you know the Naked Truth about "Covid19" and "vaccines" subject to any "genius" at Popperian Falsification that may come out of the woodwork and rebut and/or refute the assertions of some of the finest independent minds in the world in virology, infectious diseases, pulmonary critical care, immunology, epidemiology, microbiology, medicine, law etc including two Nobel Prize winners and one Nobel prize nominee whose work is reported in this book, and does so via the website below contact email address. Furthermore, ensures that the refutation/rebuttal research work is presented with fully authenticated data driven actualities, not silly 'conspiracy theories' i.e. the CIA at their very profound and erudite best; Website: https://covid19compensation2022.com/,) (that won't happen!); then **<u>you might start to consider what to do next.</u>**

[Note: **Sir Karl Popper**, The Falsification Principle, proposed by Karl Popper, is a way of demarcating science from non-science. It suggests that for a theory to be considered scientific it must be able to be tested and **conceivably** proven false. For example, the hypothesis that "all swans are white," can be falsified by observing a black swan. This little piece of wisdom assumes that the perception of the observing perceiver is infallible, which it is certainly not!]

Let's Outline all those Persons whose Circumstances are Most Probably Applicable to Compensation

CIRCUMSTANCES FOR COMPENSATION

Body Circumstances	**Possible Resolution**	**Reason for Compensation**	**Success Possibility**
1. Not Vaccinated	Compensation	UK NHS stated they could provide vaccinations for Covid19. Neither Covid19 nor vaccinations actually exist therefore they could not so provide. Note 1. 2.	0% to nominal. The logic is perfectly valid. This misinformation to the general public caused the public to waste a lot of time and money and they were put to unnecessary inconvenience.
2. Vaccinated	Compensation	Covid19 vaccines are not true vaccines and are harmful to humans. Note 2. 3.	Up to 100%. Compensation dependent upon the degree of harm suffered i.e. mild adverse effects to the extreme of limb amputation to death. Depending on specific "vaccine" toxicity.
Mind (Emotional) Circumstances	**Possible Resolution**	**Reason for Compensation**	**Success Possibility**
1. Vaccinated	Compensation	Undue stress and worry	Up to 100%. Compensation
2. Loss of Income	Compensation	Undue stress and worry	Up to 100%. Compensation

Note 1:
Proof of the existence of the SARS-CoV-2 virus by research describing the isolation of the SARS-CoV-2 virus aka COVID-19 in human beings, by scientific analysis of samples taken directly from a diseased patient, where the patient samples were not first combined with any other source of genetic material. Note: The word "isolate" means: a thing (SARS-CoV-2/COVID-19) is separated from all other material surrounding it. I am not requesting information where so-called "isolation" of SARS-CoV-2 refers to: - the culturing of

something, or - the performance of an amplification test (PCR), or - the sequencing of something. The research study methodology may require the use of Koch Postulates.

This Note 1 above requirement has never been satisfied.

Note 2:
Luc Montagnier, Nobel laureate in medicine for discovering HIV et al.

Quote:

*'**These "vaccines" are poisons. They are not real vaccines.** The mRNA allows its message to be transcribed throughout the body, uncontrollably. No one can say for each of us where these messages will go. This is therefore a terrible unknown.'*

Note 3:
Luc Montagnier, Nobel laureate in medicine for discovering HIV et al.

Quote:

*'**These "vaccines" are poisons. They are not real vaccines.** The mRNA allows its message to be transcribed throughout the body, uncontrollably. No one can say for each of us where these messages will go. This is therefore a terrible unknown.'*

Andreas Kalcker the world-renowned biophysicist has discovered that the vaccines contain large amounts of **graphene oxide** (up to 95%). He warns that the graphene oxide injected into humans is **altering their electromagnetic field**, which **disrupts the normal functioning of their organs. Please refer to horrific video below showing fibrous vein clots from "vaccines", caused by spike protein:**

Ref: https://covid19compensation2022.com/HOT-NEWS

CIRCUMSTANCES FOR COMPENSATION

Employment/ Business Circumstances	Possible Resolution	Reason for Compensation	Success Possibility
1. Placed on Furlough	Personal Compensation	Loss of Income	Up to 100% compensation
2. Lockdown	Personal Compensation	Loss of Income	Up to 100% compensation
3. Lockdown	Business Compensation	Partial Closure of Business & Loss of Income	Up to 100% compensation
4. Lockdown	Business Compensation	Full Business Closure & Full Loss of Income	Up to 100% compensation

In consideration of the fact that it has been scientifically proven by the finest independent scientific, medical, and legal minds in the world that:

1. "Sars-Cov2" does not exist and has never existed – In reality - HIV spike proteins
2. Ergo "Covid19" does not exist and has never existed – In reality -HIV spike proteins
3. "Covid19" "vaccines" do not exist and have never existed – not true vaccines - Note 3 above

then compensation should be in order.

How to Seek Compensation – A Guide
~ Form Your Own Action Group Association ~

1. Select your compensation path(s) as defined in the tables above.
2. Find people in your family, friends, place of employment, locality, clubs, the pub, 'A Stand in The Park' etc who have experienced "Covid19" "vaccination" issues as per your selection in point 1. above.

   Note: A Stand in the Park UK website:
   https://www.astandinthepark.org/uk/

   Note: A Stand in the Park Worldwide Website:
   https://www.astandinthepark.org/
3. From 2. above form a group and a committee (an association). Give the group a name. Form a committee of 3 to 6 people. Form a formal legal association.
4. It may be preferable to create a Limited Company and register it at Companies House. This may provide greater legal protection. Solicitor will advise.
5. Elect officers with at least a Chairman, Secretary, Treasurer the remainder being committee members. The Chairman chairs the meetings, the Secretary calls the meeting and takes the meeting minutes and distributes them, the Treasurer opens the bank account and handles the Association's financial affairs.
6. Define the Association's 'Mission Statement' – what you are trying to achieve and any appropriate protocols.
7. On one side of A4 define your issue and your target end goal.
8. Create an appropriate domain name for your Association and simple website explaining your 'Mission Statement' etc. A domain name and a year subscription to a self-build website costs c. £150 per annum. i.e. WordPress, 123Reg etc
9. For simplicity use website builders that have templates – no coding required i.e., 123Reg, WordPress etc. see below:

   https://www.123-reg.co.uk/website-builder/

   https://wordpress.org/

   It may be simplest to create your domain name with the same company that you use for your website builder.

10. Create social media accounts: Facebook, Twitter etc as appropriate.
11. Build as large an on-line following as you deem necessary.
12. Choose your legal strategy – Medical Negligence may be a good place to start
13. Approach no-win no fee, direct access Barristers and/or Solicitors
14. Discuss with your Barristers or Solicitors a strategy – it might be civil medical negligence or criminal medical negligence or both or something else.
15. If you require financing, investigate crowd financing options.

    Examples of Crowd Funding Sites:

    https://www.crowdfunder.co.uk/

    https://www.gofundme.com/ - Low Transaction Fees only.

16. If you use crowdfunding, you may be able expand your network through the funding methodology.
17. It may be preferable to seek compensation from the Pharmaceutical Industry. Although the industry is **supposedly** indemnified up to only £120,000 per case by the UK Government that ONLY applies to ***"unforeseen complications".***
18. It may be also preferable, to have your solicitors, barristers, advocates etc and any other professionals working for you have copies of this book. They can confirm the facts by contacting the experts (whose contributions to this book are cited) concerned if necessary. Some of the experts have already sworn under oath that their research papers, interviews, video presentations etc. are the truth, whole truth and nothing but the truth but if specific swearing may be required for specific regional legislation, then the Editor is certain of their assistance in this regard. **They all want to stop this evil, more than most!**
19. **Don't even think of giving up.**
20. **DO NOT GIVE UP**

Note:

The UK government announced that it had granted Pfizer legal indemnity protecting the American pharmaceutical company from civil lawsuits due to any **unforeseen complications** arising from problems with its **"COVID-19 vaccine"**. The special legal indemnity was the result of an emergency government **consultation** in September 2020, when the UK Department of Health & Social Care determined that changes to civil liability were necessary to better facilitate the widespread use of a "COVID-19" "vaccine" in Britain.

Ref: https://www.jurist.org/news/2020/12/uk-government-grants-pfizer-civil-legal-indemnity-for-covid-19-vaccine/

Quote: ***'granted Pfizer legal indemnity protecting the American pharmaceutical company from civil lawsuits due to any unforeseen complications arising from problems with its COVID-19 vaccine'***

The key words here are: ***'civil lawsuits', 'unforeseen complications' and 'Covid-19 "vaccine"'.***

Legally, the word "vaccine" is very important, because the finest independent scientific minds in the world state that these products are not true vaccines. See Luc Montagnier and Dr Michael McDowell. For full details see Chapters 6 and 7.

There is NO Government indemnity protection for Pfizer, Moderna etc: for criminal lawsuits, foreseen complications, nor "vaccines" that are Bioweapons/Chemical Weapons and not true vaccines at all. There is also no indemnity protection for breaking common law, civil laws or criminal laws.

Dr Reiner Fuellmich, international anti-corporate corruption trial lawyer has publicly stated that he considers because of the fact that these criminals knew exactly what they were doing, and it was all pre-planned and premeditated by them, the compensation awards are likely to be **punitive** against the perpetrators. **The damages may be in the order of millions of pounds per case.**

It is reported that Pfizer were making US$213M PER DAY for a period during the "Covid19" PLAN'demic. Their stock price essentially doubled from US$29.7 24th March 2020 to a peak at US$58.9 on 31st December 2021.

Ref: https://duckduckgo.com/?q=pfizer+share+price+2020+-+2022&atb=v344-1&ia=stock – select last 5 years

Pfizer total assets for the quarter ending September 30, 2022 were **$195.350B**, a **9.02% increase** year-over-year.

Ref: https://www.macrotrends.net/stocks/charts/PFE/pfizer/total-assets

Moderna total assets for the quarter ending September 30, 2022 were **$26.056B**, a **24.53% increase** year-over-year.

Ref: https://www.macrotrends.net/stocks/charts/MRNA/moderna/total-assets

They are therefore "Good for The Money!!" As are all companies involved in this sordid business.

Prof. Michel Chussodovsky - Professor of Economics

Quote:

'Covid19 'pandemic'* [is the] *most serious social-economic crisis in History…' 'Based on false statistics, 193 countries ordered to close down their economies...' 'the* [Covid19] *'pandemic' is economic warfare…' '*[Pfizer] *"vaccines" programmes were homicide up to* 28th *February 2022, after that date,* [Pfizer] *had their data and therefore their "vaccines" programmes became murder…'

Homicide [unlawful killing] occurs when a person kills another person. A homicide requires only a volitional act or omission that causes the death of another, and thus a homicide may result from accidental, reckless, or negligent acts even if there is no intent to cause harm.

Murder is the killing of another person without justification or excuse, especially the crime of killing a person with malice, **aforethought** or with **recklessness manifesting extreme indifference to the value of human life**.

Pfizer and the others, did they not manifest extreme indifference to the value of human life?

As Prof. Michel Chussodovsky - Professor of Economics, states above, this was **murder!**

CLAIMS

You may claim damages for bodily harm, emotional harm, or financial harm.

CORONA ACCOUNTABILITY (Covid19) 2022 would strongly recommend that you pursue your claim against the Pharmaceutical Companies, in particular the company that provided your "vaccine". The company name, the lot number and batch number of the vaccine will be recorded on your health records. Your GP should be able to provide you with this information. You will require all the information that is stored on this matter. Issue the claim on the CEO or equivalent of the company at the company's registered address. The potential harm of your vaccine should be on the database linked on the CORONA ACCOUNTABILITY (Covid19) 2022 website:

https://covid19compensation2022.com/

Click on the syringe image on the home page and go to the website 'How Bad is My Batch':

https://howbadismybatch.com/ [Direct access to 'How Bad is My Batch' website]

When making your claim whether bodily injury, emotional (mind) injury or financial injury you should set out your case as follows:

Bodily Injury

Briefly describe, preferably typed on one sheet of A4 paper, your health condition immediately prior to the "Covid19" harm, or "Vaccine" harm incurred (or both!), your condition during the harm, the length of the harm, treatments for its cure, your condition once the cure had its full or partial effect. You should include your full name, DOB, home address, email address and phone number for contact. Also include witness statements and the names, NHS addresses and registration numbers of any NHS doctors that you dealt with in this process. Further include the names and addresses of any health practitioners who assisted you who were not in the NHS system. The General Medical Council GMC will provide the registration numbers for all doctors registered with them in UK. You then have to hand a working document reference that you can present to solicitors/barristers etc.

In consideration that the NHS has been ostensibly entirely complicit, or they are totally ignorant of that that they should not be, (which constitutes professional negligence) in the mass murder of people under "Covid19"/"vaccines" as described by these world experts:

Luc Montagnier (Nobel Prize winner):

'These "vaccines" are poisons. They are not real vaccines.

Kary Mullis (Nobel Prize winner):

'It* [PCR test] *does not tell you if you are sick' [It is not a diagnostic tool for anything!]

Dr Zelenko (Nobel Prize nominee):

'the "COVID"/"Vaccination" procedures are 'Crimes against Humanity' and 1st Degree Murder'

Dr Reiner Fuellmich International Anti-Corporate Corruption Trial Lawyer (Germany/USA) Cofounder 'Corona Investigative Committee' and Founder 'International Crime Investigative Committee' 'ICIC':

'New evidence from USA Government "vaccine" Adverse Event Reporting System 'VAERS' data, shows that Big Pharma is coordinating between their companies, on a rationalised premeditated deliberate basis, the distribution of toxic* [Covid19] *"vaccines" that main and kill people.'

'Mass Murder, Crimes Against Humanity' ["Covid19" paradigm]

then it may be wise to seek cures for any bodily harm from "Covid19" and/or "Covid19" "vaccines" from persons that are **not associated** with this "organisation" the UK NHS.

The UK NHS is part of the problem hence what validity does this noble institution have to be part of the solution?

Mind (Emotional) Injury

I doubt if there were many people in the UK who did not see the immensely sad and disturbing reports and photographs in the press and media of elderly people in "care" homes, laid out on their DEATH BEDS not being able to be close to, and hug, their loved ones during the lockdown farce. Indeed, there were reports of the elderly being obliged to DIE ALONE whilst their closest family breathed on separation windowpanes and their tears dripped down those cold 'panes (pains) of heartless separation' like flood water down some *'drizzling drain of destitute despair'*.

This is outrageous and cannot go unaccounted for.

Whilst these poor peoples' hearts bled to a lonely death, to die of heartbreak, Boris Johnson (King Clown) was partying in Downing Street "like 1999" (Prince-official video below) like the selfish, unfeeling idiot that he is and always will be.

Would Johnson have the courage to DIE ALONE?

Ref: https://www.youtube.com/watch?v=rblt2EtFfC4

As above:

Briefly describe, preferably typed on one sheet of A4 paper, your emotional health condition immediately prior to the "Covid19" harm, or "Vaccine" harm incurred (or both!), your condition during the harm, the length of the harm, treatments for its cure, your condition once the cure had its full or partial effect. You should include your full name, DOB, home address, email address and phone number for contact. Also include witness statements and the names, NHS addresses and registration numbers of any NHS doctors that you dealt with in this process. Further include the names and addresses of any health practitioners who assisted you who were not in the NHS system. The General Medical Council GMC will provide the registration numbers for all doctors registered with them in UK. You then have to hand a working document reference that you can present to solicitors/barristers etc.

In consideration that the NHS has been ostensibly entirely complicit, or they are totally ignorant of that that they should not be, (which constitutes professional negligence) in the mass murder of people under "Covid19"/"vaccines" as described by the world experts then it may be wise to seek cures for any bodily harm from "Covid19" and/or "Covid19" "vaccines" from persons that are **not associated** with this "organisation" the UK NHS.

The UK NHS is part of the problem hence what validity does this noble institution have to be part of the solution? Refer to all of Chapter 19 and in particular the section entitled

'The Most Irresponsible Violations of the Hippocratic Oath in UK Medical History'

which clearly demonstrates that the UK General Medical Council GMC and the National Health Service NHS knew nothing about the truth of "SarCov2" and even less about the "vaccines". There must surely be a case for widespread criminal prosecutions for this complete and total negligence of care for their patients.

Financial Injury

Again, briefly describe, preferably typed on one sheet of A4 paper, your financial circumstances immediately prior to the "Covid19" harm, or "Vaccine" harm induced or the harm induced by the farcical "Lockdowns" that emanated from "SarsCov2"/"Covid19" (that do not, nor never have existed), and your losses throughout the almost two years of "Lockdown" (March 2020-December 2021 – Government Report) utter stupidity. Have your financial adviser or accountant provide these figures and sign their authenticity. It is imperative that there can be shown a direct causality between "Covid19"/"vaccines"/"Lock downs" and consequential loss of income. This data will be very clear in those industry sectors that suffered the most from this irresponsibility i.e.

Airlines, Hotels, Restaurants & Food Service, Fitness (Gym) Centres, Beauty & Personal Care, Sports & Performing Arts, Film Music and Entertainment Theatres, Retail

Almost all sectors of the United Kingdom will see their output shrink considerably in the second quarter of 2020, due to the Coronavirus (COVID-19) pandemic and the lockdown measures enforced by the government. Education will be the most affected sector, seeing output decline by 90 percent, while accommodation and food services will shrink by 85 percent.

Ref: https://www.statista.com/statistics/1111177/coronavirus-uk-output-losses-by-sector/

Financial compensation for these sectors, in particular: Airlines, Hotels, Restaurants & Food Service, Fitness (Gym) Centres, Beauty & Personal Care, Sports & Performing Arts, could run into £Ms per litigation action

"Covid19" Pharmaceutical Companies in UK

ASTRAZENECA PLC
Company number **02723534**

Registered Office Address:

1 Francis Crick Avenue, Cambridge Biomedical Campus, Cambridge, United Kingdom, CB2 0AA

Write to: **Pascal Soriot** Executive Director and Chief Executive Officer at the above address with copy to **Leif Johansson** Non-Executive Chair of the Board at the above address.

MODERNA BIOTECH UK LIMITED
Company number **11990046**

Registered Office Address:

54 Portland Place, London, England, W1B 1DY

Write to: **Brian Taylor Sandstrom** Secretary/Director at the above address with copy to **Cristoph Brackmann** Director at the same address.

PFIZER LIMITED
Company number **00526209**

Registered Office Address:

Pfizer Limited, Ramsgate Road, Sandwich, Kent, CT13 9NJ

Write to: **Susan Rienow** UK Managing Director and Country Manager at the above address and copy **Ben Osborn** Regional President Pfizer Hospital Business Unit for International Developed Markets at the same address.

These employment positions were announced on 11th February 2022 with Susan Rienow taking over from Ben Osborn the previous UK Managing Director and Country Manager.

CORONA ACCOUNTABILITY (Covid19) 2022 would recommend that those persons named above, each buy a copy of this book and seek the best legal advice in the world. They are going to need it, but they will lose. It is suggested that by 2030 BIG PHARMA will be small pharma and broken up into a highly regulated set of public/private organisations that will see no evil, hear no evil, do no evil. Some of the senior management of these psychopathic Big Pharma companies may be detained under His Majesty's Pleasure. So be it!

Fortune favours the brave, but not the stupid nor reckless. These people have not only been stupid, reckless, and morally moronic, they have been **EVIL to a degree not seen before in the entire History of the species homo sapiens.**

Please be our guest – get after them and get your JUSTICE you deserve.

NO WIN NO FEE Solicitors UK – some examples

Possible no win no fee UK solicitors that cover Medical Negligence are:

Medical Negligence Assist

UK Medical Negligence Claims - Free Advice & 100% No Win No Fee

Ref: https://www.medicalnegligenceassist.co.uk/

Irwin Mitchell

Medical Negligence Claims

Ref: https://www.irwinmitchell.com/personal/medical-negligence

Slater & Gordon **No Win No Fee Possibilities**

Medical Negligence Claims
If you've suffered an injury or illness as a result of medical negligence, you may be entitled to compensation. It doesn't matter whether you were in the UK or abroad, we're here to help. Talk to us about the possibility of making a medical negligence claim under a No Win No Fee agreement.

Ref: https://www.slatergordon.co.uk/medical-negligence/

United Solicitors

Medical Negligence Claims
At United Solicitors, a team of medical negligence solicitors in Manchester deal with all types of clinical negligence claims on 100% No Win No Fee basis.

Ref: https://www.united-solicitors.co.uk/medical-negligence/

Slee Blackwell Solicitors

Slee Blackwell medical negligence team is recommended by The Legal 500

We specialise in No Win, No Fee for medical negligence claims nationwide.

In most cases we suggest that you take out insurance to cover any expenses of the case, such as court fees or medical experts' fees. This insurance also covers your opponent's costs in circumstances where you could become legally responsible for paying them.

Ref: https://www.sleeblackwell.co.uk/

Other Solicitors who have been involved in "Covid19"

PJH Law **No Win No Fee Solicitors**

https://pjhlaw.co.uk/

The Good Law Project

https://goodlawproject.org/ - **home page**

https://goodlawproject.org/?s=covid – **"Covid19"**

Legal Fees & Court Fees

If you win
Typically, if you win your case, then your legal fees and court fees are paid by the losing defendant. You may well have to pay the court fees in advance so you will need to budget for that temporary expenditure. The solicitor can advise on these fees that will probably be case dependent.

If you lose
One would imagine that it would be difficult to lose a case since "SarsCov2"/"Covid19" have been proven to be non-existent, throughout this book and elsewhere. **It is incumbent upon the defendant to prove otherwise!** Secondly, it is well known, amongst intelligent, independent thinkers that the "vaccines" are not true vaccines, but are mRNA genome treatments, carrying to various levels of toxicity, spike proteins, graphene oxide and other toxic substances and are poisonous and dangerous.

Note: "intelligent, independent thinkers" excludes with regards to "SarsCov2"/"Covid19" and the associated "vaccines" any person in the world who is employed by the blockheads who run the global mainstream media; that means in UK: 'The Times' 'The Sunday Times' 'The Sunday Telegraph' 'The Observer' 'The Sunday Express' 'The Daily Telegraph' 'The Guardian' 'The Sun' 'The Daily Express' 'The Mirror' 'Private Eye' 'The Spectator' 'The New Statesman' 'The Daily Slut' 'BBC' all other television channels; the whole gamut of intellectually moribund drivel that goes as 'newspapers'.

These people are either stupid, paid off, or under the thumb of certain organisations and their repressive directives. Or perhaps all of those above.

If you do happen to lose, then you will be obliged to pay the court fees, the defendant's fees and possibly compensation to the defendant. This issue may be fully covered by taking out a onetime insurance policy as mentioned above.

An alternative to an insurance policy is crowd funding.

Crowd Funding – Class Actions

Crowdfunding is the practice of funding a project or venture by raising money from a large number of supportive people, typically via the internet. Crowdfunding is a form of crowdsourcing and alternative finance. In 2015, over US$34 billion was raised worldwide by crowdfunding.

Although similar concepts can also be executed through mail-order subscriptions, benefit events, and other methods, the term crowdfunding refers to internet-mediated registries. This modern crowdfunding model is generally based on three types of actors – the project initiator(s) who proposes the idea or project to be funded, individuals or groups who support the idea, and a moderating organization that brings the parties together to launch the idea.

Ref: https://en.wikipedia.org/wiki/Crowdfunding

UK – Some Crowd Funding Sites

(Not all are suitable for litigation)

Ref: https://www.easyship.com/blog/best-crowdfunding-sites

1. **Crowdcube** https://www.crowdcube.com/
2. **Kickstarter** https://www.kickstarter.com/
3. **Syndicate Room** https://www.syndicateroom.com/
4. **Indiegogo** https://www.indiegogo.com/
5. **GoFundme** https://www.gofundme.com/
6. **JustGiving** https://www.justgiving.com/
7. **Crowdfunder** https://www.crowdfunder.co.uk/
8. **Seedrs** https://www.seedrs.com/
9. **Funding Circle** https://www.fundingcircle.com/uk/
10. **Fundable** https://www.fundable.com/

Perhaps 6.JustGiving or 7.Crowdfunder may be the most appropriate.

CLASS ACTIONS

A **class action**, also known as a **class-action lawsuit**, **class suit**, or **representative action**, is a type of lawsuit where one of the parties is a group of people who are represented collectively by a member or members of that group. The class action originated in the

United States and is still predominantly a US phenomenon, but Canada, as well as several European countries with civil law, have made changes in recent years to allow consumer organizations to bring claims on behalf of consumers or other claimants.

A class action enables claims with common issues to be resolved in a single case. Proceedings can be brought by one claimant on its own behalf and as a representative of others. The representative's proceeding defines the group or 'class', and automatically includes all claims within that class unless a class member expressly opts out. It may be possible to crowd fund a case and use the contacts from the crowd funding to gain become, at least in part, the support for the class action. Gaining the traction for the numbers of companies supporting a class action/crowd funding may be best achieved by using industrial/business societies, business institutes, trade unions, trade associations, regional groups, clubs, societies, etc. Say your sector is 'Hospitality' then you may use, in part HOSPITALITY NET:

Ref: https://www.hospitalitynet.org/organization/17015097.html

Which interestingly stated that **Two years of Covid did £115bn damage to UK hospitality industry** – Ref as above.

Pfizer, alone have estimated assets of US$195Bn which means they Pfizer should be able to cover the loss damage to the entire UK hospitality sector – just!

Whether one may use a class action itself would depend on the circumstances of the particular lawsuit.

Harbour Litigation Funding may be able to assist with funding. From their website:

Harbour Litigation Funding

When we fund individuals or corporate claimants, we can pay all the legal fees and disbursements over the lifetime of the claim. In exchange, when the claim succeeds and damages are awarded, we receive a pre-agreed share of the amount recovered. If the claim does not succeed, our funding is written off, and the loss is Harbour's alone. Alternatively, there are other Harbour **products** which are available to meet your funding needs.

Harbour is one of the world's leading funders of group and class actions. We fund claims involving securities, shareholders, data breaches, consumer claims, mass torts, competition disputes, and more. We know where the risks arise, and what obstacles you are likely to face.

Harbour supports those who suffer loss or damage as a result of the negligence of their professional advisers. Learn how we help shareholders, creditors, insolvency practitioners and others to seek redress.

Ref: https://harbourlitigationfunding.com/

CHAPTER 18

LESSONS FOR HISTORY THE "PANDEMIC" WAS PLANNED

Ref: https://stopworldcontrol.com/proof/

23 Reasons Explain Why The "Pandemic" Was Planned

[If anyone can refute these arguments please do so through the website contact page:https://covid19compensation2022.com/]

1. Thousands of medical doctors around the world are calling the pandemic a global crime, a world dictatorship with a sanitary excuse.

   World Doctors Alliance:
   'Greatest Crime in History'

   They reveal how the pandemic is the greatest crime in history and offer solid scientific evidence for this claim.

   'The Corona panic is a play. It's a scam. A swindle. It's high time we understood that we're in the midst of a global crime.'

   'Covid-19 is a false pandemic created for political purposes. This is a world dictatorship with a sanitary excuse. We urge doctors, the media and political authorities to stop this criminal operation by spreading the truth.'

2. In the years prior to "COVID-19", the entire world suddenly began distributing hundreds of millions of PCR test kits for "COVID-19".

   The new "COVID-19" "disease" appeared in China towards the end of 2019. That's why it was named "COVID-19", which is an acronym for "**Corona Virus Disease 2019".** Data from the World Integrated Trade Solution, (World Bank) however, shows something astonishing:

   In 2017 and 2018, hundreds of millions of COVID-19 Test Kits were distributed worldwide.

   Let this sink in for a second: literally hundreds of millions of "COVID-19" test kits were exported and imported, all over the world, during 2017 and 2018. *Hundreds of millions!*

   [If the entire world circa 195 countries were in the business of exporting and importing "Covid19" Test Kits in 2017, then they were probably designed and approved in 2015 and manufactured in 2016. **"2015 is a full 5 years before the first "Covid19" break out at the end of December 2019!!]**

This baffling data was discovered by someone on **September 5, 2020**, who posted it on social media. It went viral all over the world. The next day, on **September 6,** the WITS suddenly changed the original label 'COVID-19' into the vague term 'Medical Test Kits'. But their cover up came too late: this critical information was uncovered and is being revealed by millions worldwide.

If there is anyone in the world who can explain these FACTS and PROVE that there is a rational explanation OTHER than the "pandemic" was planned, then let the world know by writing to our website: https://covid19compensation2022.com/ and CORONA ACCOUNTABILITY (Covid19) 2022 will dutifully inform the world of the explanation.

3. In 2013, a researcher predicted that a global pandemic with a coronavirus would occur in 2020. He knew this because of personal investigation of so-called 'conspiracy theories'.

   In 2008 a Worldwide lockdown was ***predicted***

   The author and investigator Robin de Ruiter predicted in 2008 that there would be a global lockdown. **He said the purpose of this would be to create a new world of authoritarian control.** Because much of what he wrote back in 2008 is now happening right in front of our eyes, this book has been republished.

4. In 2017, Anthony Fauci *guaranteed* a surprise outbreak of an infectious disease during the first term of the Trump administration. In 2017, Anthony Fauci made a very strange prediction, with an even stranger certainty. With complete confidence, Fauci guaranteed that **during the first term of President Trump,** a surprise outbreak of an infectious disease would surely happen. Here's what he said:

   'There is NO QUESTION there is going to be a challenge for the coming administration in the arena of infectious diseases.'

   'There will be a SURPRISE OUTBREAK.'

   'There's NO DOUBT in anyone's mind about this.'

5. Just before the global coronavirus pandemic began, in December 2019, Bill Gates organized a global coronavirus pandemic exercise on 18th October 2019, called **'Event 201'**.

'Event 201'

Ref: https://www.centerforhealthsecurity.org/our-work/exercises/event201/

Bill Gates is the world's number one "vaccine" dealer, who has doubled his fortune of 50 billion dollars to over 100 billion simply by dealing in "vaccines" all over the world. He has said that this has been his 'best business investment' ever. A few months before the outbreak, Bill Gates organized an event in New York City called **Event 201**. Guess what the event was all about? It was a ***'coronavirus pandemic exercise'***.

Bill Gates quote: ***'I'm particularly excited about what the next year could mean for one of the best buys in global health: vaccines.'***

6. Also shortly before the outbreak, the Global Preparedness Monitoring Board told the world to be ready for a coronavirus pandemic.

   In September 2019 - also right before the outbreak - the Global Preparedness Monitoring Board 'GPMB' released a report titled 'A World At Risk'.

   It stressed the need to be prepared for... a coronavirus outbreak!

   On the cover of the report is the picture of a coronavirus and people wearing face masks.

7. In 2018, the Institute for Disease Modelling predicted a global pandemic with a flu virus, originating in China in the area of Wuhan.

   In 2018, The Institute for Disease Modelling produced a video depicting **a flu virus (which is a coronavirus) originating in China, from the area of Wuhan, and spreading all over the world**, killing millions. They called it **'A Simulation For A Global Flu Pandemic.'** That is exactly what happened two years later.

8. In 2018, Bill and Melinda Gates announced that in the coming years there would be a global pandemic of an engineered virus.

   In 2018, Bill Gates publicly announced that *'**a global pandemic was on its way** that could wipe out 30 million people'*. He said this would ***'probably happen during the next decade'***.

   Melinda Gates added that an **engineered virus** is humanity's greatest threat, and also assured that this would hit humanity **in the coming years.**

9. The "coronavirus" "SARS-CoV-2" may have been created in the Bio Safety Lab Level 4 in Wuhan, which received millions of dollars from Anthony Fauci.

   Where did the virus come from? One of the world's leading experts in bioweapons is **Dr. Francis Boyle.** He is convinced it originated from a bioweapon lab in Wuhan - the Bio Safety Lab Level 4.

   This facility is specialized in the development of... coronaviruses!
   They work with existing viruses to weaponize [gain of function] them - meaning they make them far more dangerous, to be used as a biological weapon.

   Now comes the interesting part: in 2015 Anthony Fauci gave this very lab, Wuhan - the Bio Safety Level 4 Lab US$3.7 million dollars!!

10. Several movies have depicted the coronavirus pandemic with great detail and have even mentioned hydroxychloroquine as the cure.

    Predictive programming (through mostly the film industry) is the process of informing the population about events that are soon to occur. [The mainstream media are constantly involved in this psychological process, partly perhaps, without being aware that they are.] In past years, several movies and television series have been produced about... a global coronavirus pandemic!

The film *'Dead Plague'* depicts a global pandemic with a coronavirus, and even mentions hydroxychloroquine as the cure.

Another film called ***'Contagion'*** shows how a coronavirus spreads globally - with social distancing, face masks, lockdowns, washing of hands, etc. as a result.

Literally everything we see now, is predicted in detail in these movies.

11. A comic book produced by the European Union depicts a virus spreading worldwide. The crisis is solved by implementing totalitarian medical tyranny.

    In 2012, a strange comic book was produced by the European Union, **for distribution among their employees only.** The title of the comic is ***'INFECTED'***, and it shows **a new virus originating in a Chinese lab and spreading across the world.** The solution for this pandemic is outlined in the comic book: globalists enforce one global health plan. This means:

    No more medical freedom,

    but medical tyranny by globalist entities.

    One of the quotes of the comic book reads:

    'The safety measures that followed made our existence totally unbearable.'

12. The Summer Olympics in 2012 presented in their opening show the scenario of a pandemic from a coronavirus.

    During the opening show of the Summer Olympics in 2012, a coronavirus pandemic was played out for the eyes of the entire world.

    Dozens of hospital beds, large numbers of nurses becoming puppets of a controlling system, death lurking about, a demonic giant rising up over the world, and the whole theatre was lit up in such a way that, seen from the sky, it looked like a coronavirus.

    Why did the Olympic Games show a coronavirus pandemic, in their opening show?

13. The investigative journalist **Harry Vox** predicted in 2014 that a global pandemic would be created so the 'ruling class' could implement a higher level of authoritarian control.

    In 2014, Harry Vox predicted a planned global pandemic, and explained why the 'ruling class' would do such thing:

    'They will stop at nothing to complete their toolkit of control. One of the things that had been missing from their toolkit was quarantines and curfews. The plan is to get hundreds of thousands of people infected with it and <u>create the next phase of control.</u>'

14. The investigative journalist Anthony Patch predicted a global pandemic with a man-made virus - that would be used to force a DNA-altering vaccine on humanity.

    During an interview in 2014, this researcher predicted the following:

    'They will release a man-made 'coronavirus'. As a result, the people will demand a vaccine to protect them. This vaccine will add a third strand of DNA to a person's body, essentially making them a hybrid. Once a person is injected, almost immediately their DNA undergoes a transformation. This genetic change will cause people to lose the ability to think for themselves, without them even being aware this has happened. Thus, they can be controlled more easily, to become slaves for the elite.'

    Of course, that sounds insane - and it is insane indeed. Yet we have to realize that this professional investigator is no fool. He has invested years of research into this subject, and this is what he has discovered during this time. [Indeed, Yuval Harari advisor to Klaus Schwab WEF has endorsed this insanity on numerous occasions – see below:

    Yuval Harari advisor to Klaus Schwab WEF World Economic Forum

    "Governments and Corporations can hack Human Beings... Soul, Spirit, Free Will - in humans, that's over!!!"

    Ref: https://www.youtube.com/watch?v=NV0CtZga7qM

15. Dr. Carrie Madej has studied DNA and vaccines for decades, and her research has shown that the plan is to use the "COVID-19" vaccine to start the process of **transhumanism**:

    reprogramming the human DNA.

    Ref: https://stopworldcontrol.com/proof/

    She has made an urgent video in which she warns that there is a plan to inject humanity with very dangerous "vaccines" for "Covid-19". The purpose of these new "vaccines" will be twofold:

    A) **Reprogram our DNA and make us hybrids that are easier to control.**

    B) **Connect us to artificial intelligence through a digital vaccine ID, which will also open a whole new realm of control.**

    This medical expert says she has observed on multiple occasions how diseases were spread over populations by aircraft. For safety reasons, she is not able to share more details about this in public.

16. The CIA officer **Dr. John Coleman** studied secret societies in depth, and states that their goal is to depopulate the earth by means of organized pandemics of fatal, rapid acting diseases. Dr. John Coleman was an Intelligence Officer from the CIA who wrote a book titled ***'The Committee of 300'***. In the book, he explains how secret societies manipulate governments, health care, food industries, the media and so on. This book can be found on the website of the CIA.

One of the primary goals of the many secret societies that control governments and the media, is to depopulate the earth.

'At least 4 billion "useless eaters" shall be eliminated by the year 2050 by means of limited wars and organized epidemics of fatal, rapid acting diseases.'

17. In the state of Georgia, USA, a huge monument was erected in 1980 with ten guidelines for humanity in eight languages. The first of these 'Ten Commandments' is that humanity needs to be reduced to half a billion people.

18. **Bill Gates** said during a TED talk that new vaccines can be used to reduce the world's population by 10-15%.

    'There are now 6.7 billion people on earth and soon there will be 9 billion. However, we can reduce that number by ten to fifteen percent if we do a good job with new vaccines, health care and birth control. **[How do new vaccines and health care reduce population growth unless the "vaccines" are poisons that kill people, and the health care is not healthy and thus similarly kills people?!]**

19. The 'Health Ranger', Mike Adams, predicted years ago what we see happening now: the release of an engineered bioweapon, followed by a vaccine mandate, massive government funding for the vaccine industry and a vaccine that has been developed in record time.

    'An engineered bioweapon will be released in population centres. There will be calls for massive government funding for the vaccine industry to come up with a vaccine. Miraculously they will have a vaccine developed in record time. Everyone will be required to line up and take this vaccine shot.'

    The rest of his message is that this "vaccine" will slowly begin to kill millions - if not billions - of people over the course of a few years. It will be a kill-switch "vaccine", designed to reduce the world's population.

20. In 2010, the **Rockefeller Foundation** published the ***'Scenario for the Future***...' in which they describe a coming global pandemic that is intended to result in the implementation of authoritarian control over the people and is planned to intensify after the pandemic.

    This famous document by the Rockefeller Foundation in which everything we see happening now is literally predicted in great detail: the global pandemic, the lockdowns, the collapse of the economy and the imposing of authoritarian control.

    It's all described with terrifying accuracy... ***ten years before it happened!***

    The document is titled '**Scenario for the Future of Technology and International Development**'. It is available online.

    That says it all: '***a scenario for the future'.*** It has a chapter called '**LockStep**', in which a global pandemic is reported as if it had happened in the past, but which is **clearly intended as a rehearsal for the future.**

21. In 2020, the **Rockefeller Foundation** published a handbook on how to create this world of control, with a step-by-step guide. They state that life cannot return back to normal until the world has become **'Locked Down'** with this top-down control from authoritarian governments. Now that the announced pandemic is indeed here, the same Rockefeller Foundation has come forward with step two: **a handbook on how to implement new control systems during this pandemic.** The book reveals that only when all the required control networks are in place can the world open up again.

    These are quotes from their guide:

    'Digital apps and privacy-protected tracking software should be widely used to enable more complete contact tracking.'

    'In order to fully control the Covid-19 epidemic, we need to test the majority of the population on a weekly basis.'

    According to their ''*Scenario for the Future of Technology and International Development*', the entire world population should get a digital ID that indicates who has received all the vaccines. Without sufficient vaccinations, access to schools, concerts, churches, public transport, etc., will be denied.
    And now, as of 2020, that is exactly what Bill Gates, and many governments are calling for.

    In a leaked government video, we see a conversation between former American president **Bill Clinton and Andrew Cuomo**, the governor of the state of New York. They discuss how to set up a large control system to test the entire population and check all their contacts. They discuss how to build an army to carry out this control system.

22. We indeed are seeing that **Bill Gates** and many others worldwide are right away seizing control in unprecedented ways: by enforcing "vaccine" ID's (microchips to be implanted into people), mandating the wearing of face masks, social distancing, forced lockdowns, extreme contact tracing, and so on.

    Bill Gates also made it clear that only people who have been "vaccinated" against "Covid-19" should be allowed to travel, go to school, attend meetings and work. Digital "vaccine" ID's are already being developed and Gates has a patent on the technology that makes it possible to trace an individual's body anywhere. This technology is called WO2020-060606. In addition, Gates wants to set up a global monitoring network which will track everyone who has come into contact with "Covid-19". [Is this "man" not mad?]

    [**Here is an outline of Bill Gates patent:**
    There are many plot theories today such as beverages which produced by Coca-Cola contain the blood of Christian babies, reptiles rule the US government. Certain technological events are interpreted by prophecies in the Bible. There are some reasonable facts that cannot be denied such as the presence of the Bilderberg

Club, the CIA's MK-Ultra project, and George Soros' funding for suspicious political activities.

Patent WO / 2020/060606 relates to officially recorded facts. It was registered on March 26, 2020. It was made by Microsoft Technology Licensing LLC under the presidency of **Gates** and gained international status on April 22, 2020. **'Cryptocurrency system using body activity data'** is the title of this patent.

The online patent application can be summarized as follows: The human body activity associated with the task provided to a user can be used in the mining process of a cryptocurrency system. A server can provide a task to a user's device connected to the server. A sensor attached to the user's device or positioned within it can detect the user's body activity. Body activity data can be generated based on the attained body activity of the user. The cryptocurrency system connected to the user's device can verify whether the data generated by body activity meet the conditions set by the cryptocurrency system and can issue cryptocurrency to the user whose body activity data is verified."

In other words, thanks to the crypto money, the chip that monitors the daily physical activity of the person will be placed in the body. If the conditions are met, the person receives certain bonuses that can be spent on something.

In a detailed description of the invention, it explains how to use the device with 28 concepts.

It also provides a list of countries for which the invention is intended.]

Ref:https://proippatent.com/Infocenter/detail/47/what-is-patent-060606-microchip-and-famous-bill-gates-patent-number?lang=en

[DO NOT CLAIM THAT YOU HAVE NOT BEEN WARNED]

23. Part of this top-down control is the extreme censoring and de-platforming of literally every voice from doctors, scientists and other experts who dare to question or criticize what is happening.

Ref: https://stopworldcontrol.com/proof/

CHAPTER 19

REQUESTS FOR INFORMED CONSENT FOR "COVID19" "VACCINATION" FROM 15TH OCTOBER 2022 UK FREEDOM OF INFORMATION ACT 2000 REQUEST FOIA

The Most Irresponsible Violations of the Hippocratic Oath in UK Medical History

On 15th October 2022 the Editor of this book attended St Thomas' Hospital, Westminster Bridge Road, London for a "Covid19" "vaccination". He was shown into a small surgery and the "vaccinating" Doctor informed him that he was to receive the Pfizer "vaccination".

The Good Doctor failed to inform the editor that Pfizer were the largest criminals in USA history in 2009. Pfizer was the biggest felon in the History of USA if you denote "biggest" by the size of the criminal and civil fines imposed upon the Company, being 2.3US$Bn for fraudulent marketing of which **1.189US$Bn was a criminal fine**; quote ***'the largest criminal fine ever imposed in the United States for any matter.'***

Ref: **USA Justice Department:** Url link: https://www.justice.gov/opa/pr/justice-department-announces-largest-health-care-fraud-settlement-its-history

How's that for informed consent?

What person who lays legitimate claims to being an inherent part of the homo sapiens gene pool, would allow the bunch of the world's largest criminals to inject into their sovereign bodies, a load of untrialled junk **and** were informed that a criminally convicted company wished to go about their sordid untrialled **US$213M revenue per day** in the "Covid19" jab revenue business?

When the Doctor had completed the form filling, the Editor read the letter below out loud to the Doctor in request of information so that the editor could make an informed decision in order to give his informed consent– see Appendix II.

The entire procedure was filmed by the Editor so that a legal record could be held to perpetuity. The Editor was informed that it was not permitted to film in a hospital without permission. The Editor replied that he was not aware of that fact and that he had not seen any warning signs to that effect anywhere in the building. He then immediately ceased filming.

Professor Ian Abbs
Chief Executive
St Thomas' Hospital
Vaccination Centre 1
Westminster Bridge Road
London SE1 7EH

15th October 2022

COVID19 VACCINATION

FREEDOM OF INFORMATION ACT 2000 FOIA REQUEST 1

Thank you for your offer to vaccinate me against Covid19 [on the above date]. Before I proceed to accept your offer of Covid19 vaccination, I would like to ensure that **I am able to provide you** with **my** **informed consent.**

Please provide:

1. Proof of the existence of the SARS-CoV-2 virus by research describing the isolation of the SARS-CoV-2 virus aka COVID-19 in human beings, by scientific analysis of samples taken directly from a diseased patient, where the patient samples were not first combined with any other source of genetic material. Note: The word "isolate" means: a thing (SARS-CoV-2/COVID-19) is separated from all other material surrounding it. I am not requesting information where so-called "isolation" of SARS-CoV-2 refers to: - the culturing of something, or - the performance of an amplification test (PCR), or - the sequencing of something. The research study methodology may require the use of Koch Postulates.
2. Proof that all the vaccines approved for use in UK such as: Moderna vaccine, Oxford/AstraZeneca vaccine, Pfizer/BioNTech vaccine and any other vaccine approved for use in UK but not here listed, are all safe for human use and do not contain any graphene oxide or any other substances in any way harmful to humans.

Note that if this material requested in points 1. and 2. above is not readily available to your organization then it should be readily available from one or more of the persons on the list overleaf. **This Notice under the Freedom of Information Act 2000 is simultaneously served on the list of persons overleaf by Royal Mail.** All recipients are formally requested to reply individually, being independently causal agents in this matter of SARS-CoV-2/ COVID-19.

Recipient List	**Office** (at the time of Covid19 – 2019/2020 onwards)
Boris Johnson	**Prime Minister**
Matt Hancock	**Health & Social Care**
Nadhim Zahawi	**"Covid" "Vaccine" Deployment**
Michael Gove	**Cabinet Office**
Sajid Javid	**Health & Social Care**
Suella Braverman	**Attorney General**
Priti Patel	**Home Office**
Baroness Hallett	**Chair Covid Inquiry 2021-**
Christopher Whitty	**Chief Medical Officer/Chief Medical Advisor**
Patrick Vallance	**Chief Scientific Advisor**
June Munro Raine	**CEO MHRA** - Medicines and Healthcare Products Regulatory Agency
Charlie Massey	**CEO GMC** – General Medical Council
Amanda Pritchard	**CEO NHS** – National Health Service
Neil Ferguson	**Researcher** - Imperial College, London
Dr Gillian Ostrowski	**Medical Doctor** formerly NHS Bridge Lane Practice/South West London Covid19 Testing Centre – This FOI Request is made under this former employment
Dr Johannes Coetzee	**Medical Doctor** NHS Bridge Lane Practice
Joanne Lawson	**Practice Management** NHS Bridge Lane Practice

Your reply by email with attachments or URL links to the material requested will suffice.

END OF LETTER

[Legal Note: The UK's FREEDOM OF INFORMATION ACT 2000 FOIA is very clear.

Public authorities are required to respond to FOI requests no later than 20 working days after they were made. As of today's date, 13th December 2022 NOT ONE reply has been received from the 18 persons who were requested to provide the FOIA information. This constitutes a potential breach of law by all parties, since the total of working days now stands at 40 days, twice that that is permitted.]

Source of the information below, NHS UK website:

Ref: https://www.nhs.uk/conditions/consent-to-treatment/

*'**Consent** to treatment means a person must give permission before they receive any type of medical treatment, test or examination. This must be done on the basis of an explanation by a clinician. **Consent** from a patient is needed regardless of the procedure, whether it's a physical examination, organ donation or something else.'*

Defining consent

For consent to be valid, it must be **voluntary** and **informed**, and the person consenting must have the capacity to make the decision.

The meaning of these terms are:

- voluntary – the decision to either consent or not to consent to treatment must be made by the person, and must not be influenced by pressure from medical staff, friends or family
- informed – the person must be given all of the information about what the treatment involves, including the benefits and risks, whether there are reasonable alternative treatments, and what will happen if treatment does not go ahead
- capacity – the person must be capable of giving consent, which means they understand the information given to them and can use it to make an informed decision

It is the considered legal opinion of the Editor, that the two points above: 'informed…' and 'capacity…' **were not adhered to in any of the millions of cases of "Covid19" "vaccinations"** and as consequence all the causal agents, listed above and possibly others, are potentially liable to very serious prosecution. In consideration of the disastrous affects that these "vaccines" have had on the 75% of the UK population i.e., c. 45M people, who received c. 140Million "vaccinations" then the damages may well be punitive. Punitive is a very important legal term in this regard.

The Doctor then left the surgery and returned with a Senior Nurse. The Nurse took the letter and said that another colleague had 'The Green Book' and hence the editor assumed that the person with a copy of the Green Book would be able to provide the information required for informed consent.

Two senior persons, one a doctor the other a Service Manager, then came into the surgery and the editor was asked the reason for his visit to the "Vaccination" centre to which he answered that he wanted the information so that he could give his informed consent to the "vaccination", providing that the information provided by the NHS was conducive to doing so.

There was no reply to the two questions above, required for informed consent, provided by any member of the NHS staff involved in the discussion. The editor was then requested to promptly leave the building and was escorted off the premises by the "Service Manager".

The behaviour of all the NHS staff involved is a clear breach of the NHS document on their website showing the definition of consent which is shown above **including the terms voluntary, informed and capacity**.

Furthermore, the UK NHS is in clear breach of its duties because the NHS failed to inform the UK population of:

- informed – the person must be given all of the information about what the treatment involves, including the benefits and **risks,** whether there are **reasonable alternative treatments**, and what will happen if treatment does not go ahead

There is no information on the NHS website about these alternative treatments:

Cure No 1: Hydroxychloroquine (HCQ) + Zinc

Cure No 2: The Holistic Approach: Hydrogen Peroxide

Cure No 3: Nebulized Budesonide

Cure No 4: Ivermectin

Nor the FLCCC Prevention Guide:
FLCCC: A Guide to the Prevention of "COVID-19"

Nor the Information assisting in dealing with "Covid19" that is available on the following websites:

www.CovidPatientGuide.com – Downloadable Physician List & Guide to Home-Based COVID Treatment

www.C19Protocols.com – Two Post Vaccination Protocols, 13 Early Treatment Protocols, 4 Long Covid Protocols

www.TheCovidRemedy.com General Advice and Guidance on "Covid" Introductory Video banned by Social Media Giants

www.FlemingMethod.com/best-available-published-evidence General Advice and Guidance on "Covid"

www.StopWorldControl.com/cures Good background information. Cures used in this book.

Refer to Chapter 15 above for the full details of the above.

These alternatives, some of which were available before the creation of the poisonous "vaccines", but their existence was suppressed by world "authorities". It is not permissible for the World Health Organisation WHO to claim a "pandemic" when there are treatments already available for that which is claimed to be causing the pandemic i.e. "Covid19"

63 peer reviewed studies confirm the effectiveness of Ivermectin in treating "COVID"

Biophysicist Andreas Kalcker used chlorine dioxide to slash the daily death rate of 100 to 0, in Bolivia and was asked to treat the military, police, and politicians in several Latin

American nations. His worldwide network '**COMUSAV.com**' consists of thousands of physicians, academics, scientists, and lawyers who are promoting this effective treatment.

With several options to successfully treat COVID-19, why is there still such an outcry for a fake "vaccine"? And why is the majority of the population not even aware of the available treatments? The answer is shocking and shows once more what is going on in our world...

All over the world physicians who were successfully treating "Covid" patients, encountered the unthinkable: they were intimidated and shut down by the government.

America's Frontline Doctors informed the world about the safe and effective cures for "Covid", during their first White Coat Summit in 2020. This broadcast was viewed over twenty million times in a few hours, but then they were shut down all across the board: Facebook, YouTube, Twitter, and even their website was taken down by Squarespace the website provider platform.

See Chapter 3 above.

In consideration of the amount of harm that "Covid19" and the "Vaccines" have done as reported by the finest independent minds in the world in this book; it may be the case, that the NHS and other bodies are susceptible to serious criminal prosecution.

COVID19 VACCINATION

FREEDOM OF INFORMATION ACT 2000 FOIA REQUEST 2

Upon UK GENERAL MEDICAL COUNCIL 'GMC' Nov./Dec. 2022

And GMC reply

Dear Lawrence Wolfe-Xavier

I write further to previous correspondence which has been reallocated to me.

I can see that on 15 October 2022 the GMC was asked for:

1. *Proof of the existence of the SARS-CoV-2 virus by research describing the isolation of the SARS-CoV-2 virus aka COVID-19 in human beings, by scientific analysis of samples taken directly from a diseased patient, where the patient samples were not first combined with any other source of genetic material. Note: The word "isolate" means: a thing (SARS-CoV-2/COVID-19) is separated from all other material surrounding it. I am not requesting information where so-called "isolation" of SARS-CoV-2 refers to: - the culturing of something, or - the performance of an amplification test (PCR), or - the sequencing of something. The research study methodology may require the use of Koch Postulates.*

2. *Proof that all the vaccines approved for use in UK such as: Moderna vaccine, Oxford/AstraZeneca vaccine, Pfizer/BioNTech vaccine and any other vaccine approved for use in UK but not here listed, are all safe for human use and do not contain any graphene oxide or any other substances in any way harmful to humans.*

On 10 November 2022, my colleague Mark confirmed that the GMC held no information within the scope of your request.

Kind Regards

Matt

Matthew McCoig-Lees
Senior Information Access Officer
Information Access Team
General Medical Council
3 Hardman Street
Manchester
M3 3AW

6th December 2022

Email: matt.mccoig-lees@gmc-uk.org
Website: www.gmc-uk.org
Tel: 0161 923 6579

COVID19 VACCINATION

FREEDOM OF INFORMATION ACT 2000 FOIA REQUEST 3

Upon UK NATIONAL HEALTH SERVICE 'NHS' November 2022

And NHS reply

Dear Lawrence Wolfe-Xavier,

Thank you for your communication dated 21 November 2022.

Your exact request was:

"*Please provide:*

1. *Proof of the existence of the SARS-CoV-2 virus by research describing the isolation of the SARS-CoV-2 virus AKA COVID-19 in human beings, by scientific analysis of samples taken directly from a diseased patient, where the patient samples were not first combined with any other source of genetic material.*

Note: The word 'isolate' means: a thing (SARS-CoV-2/COVID-19) is separated from all other material surrounding it. I am not requesting information where so-called 'isolation' of SARS-CoV-2 refers to: - the culturing of something, or - the performance of an amplification test (PCR), or - the sequencing of something. The research study methodology may require the use of Koch Postulates.

2. *Proof that all the vaccines approved for use in the UK such as: Moderna Vaccine, Oxford/AstraZeneca vaccine, Pfizer/BioNTech vaccine and any other vaccine approved for use in UK but not here listed, are all safe for human use and do not contain any graphene oxide or any other substances in any way harmful to humans*."

NHS England does not hold information in relation to your request.

Yours sincerely,

Freedom of Information
Communications
Strategy Directorate
NHS England
PO Box 16738
REDDITCH
B97 9PT

25th November 2022

Tel: 0300 311 22 33
Email: england.contactus@nhs.net

NHS and UK Government "Covid19" "Vaccinations" Data – Two Samples

The NHS data detailing their "Covid19" "vaccination" programmes can be found on their website referenced below:

The [total] number of people who have had an 'Autumn Booster' vaccination for COVID-19 since the 5th September 2022, by **NHS UK is 16.596M!!**

NHS Region of Residence[3]		Total number of people who have had an Autumn Booster[5] dose to date
England[4]		16,596,732

Ref: https://www.england.nhs.uk/statistics/statistical-work-areas/covid-19-vaccinations/

UK GOVERNMENT EXECUTE 85 MILLION "Covid19" "Vaccinations" by 1st August 2021

The UK Government published on 1st August 2021:

Quote:

"Press release
More than 85 million COVID-19 vaccines administered in UK

Over 88% of adults have had a first dose and over 72% of adults have had both doses.

From:

Department of Health and Social Care, The Rt Hon Sajid Javid MP, and The Rt Hon Nadhim Zahawi MP

Published
1 August 2021"

Unquote

Ref: **https://www.gov.uk/government/news/more-than-85-million-covid-19-vaccines-administered-in-uk**

The Most Irresponsible Violations of the Hippocratic Oath in UK Medical History

From the GMC and NHS responses to Freedom of Information Requests 2 and 3 above the reader will perceive the following:

What these complete idiots are freely admitting, is that according to UK/NHS Government figures and the combined "genius" of Javid (a bus-driver's son a fact he is so pleased to announce to the world as some sort of inverted snobbery advertising slogan) and Zahawi (who is apparently perhaps not the son of a bus driver) is that 85 million+++ sadly, grossly mislead persons in UK had innocently taken these "Covid19" "vaccines" when no one in the **NHS UK nor in the GMC**, (GMC is the NHS governing body for ensuring due diligence and appropriate professional conduct) had a tinker's cuss of an idea **IF the "virus" existed nor had a tinker's wife's cuss of an idea what was in the "Covid19" "vaccines"!!!!!**

Yet abounding throughout this book are independent scientific studies that state that ***"SARS-CoV-2 virus"* does not exist, but what does exist is an HIV spike protein**. Further abounding throughout this book are independent scientific studies that state that the **"Covid19" "vaccines" do contain graphene oxide and spike proteins and that they are poisonous to human beings.**

Corona Accountability (Covid19) 2022 calls upon Baroness Hallett to get to the bottom of this matter through her Covid-19 Enquiry and bring those responsible to account.

Please refer to Appendix IV Letter to Baroness Hallett, Chair UK Covid-19 Enquiry Containing Allegations of Mass Murder and Crimes Against Humanity Dated: May 2023.

As mentioned elsewhere in this book, "Sars-Cov-2" <u>IS NOT</u> a virus!

Results of Studies by Dr Poornima Wagh PhD Santa Barbara CA, USA confirm this!

Dr Poornima Wagh, Researcher, 2 PhDs in Virology and Immunology, Santa Barbara, CA, USA

Quote:

'The Scamdemic: "Covid19" Sars-Cov-2 The Virus that Never Existed'

Dr Poornima Wagh quote:

"*There's <u>NO</u>* [nor has there ever been] *Sars-Cov-2 or Covid19 nor any variants – no Gamma, no Omicron, no Delta, no Monkey Pox – Monkey Pox is a side effect on the Pfizer/Moderna/Johnson&Johnson "vaccines""*

"Studies of true isolation* [Koch Postulates] *from April to September 2020 using tests repeated three times with 1,500 samples resulted in only debris being found! NO "Sars-Cov2/Covid19" or any other virus was found" "Studies repeated in 7 Universities – same results".

Unquote

Ref: Appendix I – Appendix 29 p76 PDF Download File

As mentioned elsewhere in this book, "Covid19" "vaccines" are poisons and they kill people!

Dr Reiner Fuellmich International Anti-Corporate Corruption Trial Lawyer (Germany/USA) Cofounder 'Corona Investigative Committee' and Founder 'International Crime Investigative Committee' 'ICIC':

Quote:

'New evidence from USA Government "vaccine" Adverse Event Reporting System 'VAERS' data, shows that Big Pharma is coordinating between their companies, on a rationalised premeditated deliberate basis, the distribution of toxic* [Covid19] *"vaccines" that main and kill people.'

'Mass Murder, Crimes Against Humanity' ["Covid19" paradigm]

Unquote

Ref: Appendix I p69, Appendix 9 PDF Download File

Luc Montagnier, Nobel laureate in medicine for discovering HIV

Quote:

'These "vaccines" are poisons. They are not real vaccines. The mRNA **[messenger RNA]** ***allows its message to be transcribed throughout the body, uncontrollably. No one can say for each of us where these messages will go. This is therefore a terrible unknown.'***

'The 3 vaccines Pfizer, AstraZeneca, Moderna contain a sequence identified by Information Technology as transformation into a prion. There is therefore a known risk to human health.'

Unquote

Ref: Appendix I – p19 PDF Download File

We Remind the Reader of the Legal Case of Mr Patrick King

As previously stated, the court case then, in effect, went from Deena Hinshaw v Mr Patrick King **to Her Majesty the Queen (Queen Elizabeth II, (Buckingham Palace, London SW1A 1AA UK)) v Mr Patrick King. In this case 'The Crown' was requested to provide material evidence to the Court that the SARS-CoV-2 "virus" had been isolated (as described above i.e. proven to exist).**

The UK Crown could not provide the evidence required to the Court!

Ref: Appendix I – p16 PDF Download File

To emphasise, **Corona Accountability (Covid19) 2022** calls upon Baroness Hallett to get to the bottom of this matter through her Covid-19 Enquiry and bring those responsible to account.

CHAPTER 20

NATURAL LAW – YOUR RIGHT TO LIFE

From the pre-Socratics onwards, and possibly before those times, Humankind has been intrigued with the Mystery of Being and has contemplated, and tried to find, answers to the big questions of Life. For the most part, it might be considered, that those quests have not been particularly successful. The persons concerned, were perhaps naïve enough to believe that their queries would result in definitive answers. If definite answers were achieved, then surely the destiny on Humankind would not have been the sorry and sordid thing that it is. Humankind has achieved many good things, and some great things such as: the outlawing of slavery, improved health, improved living conditions etc. but the sad fact is that these items should not have been so bad in the first place that there was such great need to improve them.

For all our great search for Truth, the History of Humankind is not a pretty one – Chapters 1 to 7 of the book below.

Ref:

'Save Yourself Save Us All'
'How We Can All Live Happily into the 22nd Century'
'They Unique Post Covid19 Opportunity for all Humankind'

Written by Lawrence Wolfe-Xavier ISBN10 1839755318 ISBN13 9781839755316

Ref: https://saveyourselfsaveusall.co.uk/

Here is the beginning of Chapter 7:

Chapter 7 – Family of Humankind – The Nature of Man

TRUTH begins at Infinity and ends at Eternity

The Puppet 'Masters' pull the Strings of the Puppets
but the 'Masters' have No Control over Themselves

Why is the world in such a mess? Why oh, why is the world in such a mess?

What genuine progress has Humankind made in 2,000+ years of western 'civilisation'?

2000+ years of 'civilisation' and what does the Family of Humankind have to show for all its hard work and sacrifice? What true progress have we made? We have today:

List 1. Endless war(s), global starvation, global modern slavery, global self-imposed slavery; a few very, very rich people, many many very, very poor people, many in-between people without very much – "just getting by", enormous human stupidity about climate change, over exploitation of natural resources, global terrorism, corrupt international businesses, world-wide international crime, world-wide drugs crime as a self-sufficient industry in its own 'right', global human trafficking, global corporations ostensibly beyond the reach of domestic government legislation, governments 'ruled' by the social media masses and their hysteria, technological advances outstripping legislation that cannot keep up-to-date with the technology and its social effects and consequences, internationally lead violations of domestic country democratic processes, polluted over-crowded cities, city crime and city violence, city depravation, child criminality, institutionalised paedophilia, humankind's unnecessary self-inflicted suffering, religious segregation, religious antagonism, racial tensions and antagonisms, racial sectarianism, people losing their jobs for holding perfectly intellectually valid and rational views, UK police non-impartiality publicly showing racial/ethnic bias, crass stupidity of mainstream media, intrusive surreptitious surveillance capitalism, global financial market collapses owing to capitalists selling property market junk to people who have as much chance of repaying the property 'loan' as flying to mars on a 'Boris Bike', total Covid-19 incompetence and unpreparedness particularly by the numbskulls in UK government, unprotected elderly in Care Homes resulting in their deaths owing to UK government Covid-19 total incompetence, 'inverted' moral values in favour of over-represented minorities at the expense of the genuine numerical majority, ……a UK politician leading the world into a morally repugnant war declared illegal by the United Nations, so called 'world leaders' aiding and abetting the global criminal activity of human trafficking gangs,…….the list of contemporary human idiocy must be infinite, if it is not infinite then it must be greater than infinity…

Indeed, 'the many good things, and some great things' mentioned above did not come about, for the most part, as a natural (evolutionary) consequence stemming from the natural goodness in Humankind. They came about as a 'kick-back' against the repression of the many who owned little or nothing against the few that owned everything. These 'good things/great things' for the most part, were achieved by further suffering of the many in the attempts to correct the evil of the few. Such as marches from Yarrow to London, chaining oneself to railings, riots, imprisonment etc.

The Jarrow March of 5–31 October 1936, also known as the Jarrow Crusade, was an organised protest against the unemployment and poverty suffered in the English town of Jarrow during the 1930s. The Suffragettes were part of the 'Votes for Women' campaign that had long fought for the right of women to vote in the UK. They chained themselves to railings as a form of protest and were imprisoned in Holloway Prison London where they were strapped to a chair and force fed. The Peterloo Massacre took place at St Peter's Field, Manchester, Lancashire, England, on Monday 16 August 1819. Fifteen people died when cavalry charged into a crowd of around 60,000 people who had gathered to demand the reform of parliamentary representation. There we riots in Bristol from 1793 – 2021. Earl Bertrand Russell was one of the greatest minds of the 20th century and author of 'Principia Mathematica with A. N. Whitehead. Yet, in 1918, he was sentenced to six-month imprisonment in Brixton Prison for publicly lecturing against the US joining the First World War on the side of Britain. It was the first of two sentences **Russell** would serve there. During this time, **Russell** lived in London, near the British Museum. His time here is immortalized with a blue plaque. History is littered with such examples of further suffering endured to overcome the suffering objected to.

Furthermore, today almost half the world — over three billion people live on less than US $2.50 a day. **At least 80% of humanity lives on less than US $10 a day**. More than 80 percent of the world's population lives in countries where income differentials are widening.

Ref: http://www.globalissues.org/article/26/poverty-facts-and-stats

The evil we have experienced in the past still exists today. Indeed this "Covid19" "vaccines" business perhaps outstrips all previous examples of extreme evil. Here again, we see the exploitation of the many, for the enormous advantage of, and by, the very, very few.

Let us consider the Natural Order of The Universe. It is without question, we believe, that all Life that comes into being through Natural means, is a consequential product of Nature and therefore subject to Natural Law. By 'Natural Law' we mean the rules that govern the order within the world and in the 'known' universe(s). This is what this editor calls 'The Imperfect Harmony of The Universe'. A subject he will write on, destiny permitting, in future works, which will culminate in an adequate 'proof', on the balance of probabilities, of the existence of a 'First Cause' or a 'Creator'. This essay will not in any way whatsoever be predicated on any form of religious faith. It will be based on rationalism, logic, and dialectics.

So, all Life or Beings of any manner whatsoever, that come into being, (becoming a form of life) - through Natural means, by definition, must have a right to the continuance of that life or being. This is inherent in Natural Law.

What we are observing in the case of this "Covid19" "vaccines" business, is that the diktat of Natural Law is being violated by some very low intelligence and very low sense of Ethics and Morals of very powerful, rich, and dangerous people. The problem with these people is that, apart from their lack of Ethics and Morals they have a psychological profile, over which they have little or no control, which does not permit them to be otherwise.

As we have seen with the Standard Deviation Diagram of Human Love, Empathy, Compassion page x

At the + (positive) end of 0.1% these persons one might say, are perfectly conscious and perfectly conscious of their consciousness. However, their Human Love, Empathy, Compassion is as low as those confined to institutions. This is why they can "operate" on this mass murder programme level with little or no remorse. Such a concept as remorse is not within them, similarly neither is Human Love, Empathy, Compassion.

The 0.1% of the global population, are the persons at the top of the hierarchical chain implementing the "Covid19" "vaccines" 'Great Reset' mass murder and Transhumanism program as we note below from a previous reference to this insanity.

Yuval Harari advisor to Klaus Schwab WEF World Economic Forum quote:

'Governments and Corporations can hack Human Beings...you can manipulate them in ways that were previously impossible.... Soul, Spirit, Free Will - in humans, that's over!!!'

Ref: https://www.youtube.com/watch?v=NV0CtZga7qM

Since these evil people have no comprehension of any form of higher ideal other than mere lowly materialism, then they have no concept of the Natural Law discussed. Having no concept and therefore no understanding of Natural Law and its importance, they defy it. Being what they are, they are condemned to defy it.

It is preposterous that Harari be described, which he is in the media, as some sort of philosopher; Plato, Kant, Leibniz, Schopenhauer et al would turn in their graves at the idea. It is not possible to be a philosopher without some understanding of Ethics and Morality. It is however possible to be an idiot without some understanding of Ethics and Morality. There are suspicions, that Harari spouts his Transhumanism nonsense, in part, to impress Klaus Schwab, in obedience to his 'The Great Leader' of the 'WEF'. He is also described as a 'public intellectual'. There is no such thing. There is no point in a thinker or 'intellectual' being 'public', because the 'public' are unlikely to understand a true thinker. Some people mistakenly play this game, perhaps to sell more books. Harari is an historian. He churns up the past and presents it in the present. Bravo! A past, from which, homo sapiens appear to learn very little.

Being agents of mass murder, these idiots are violating Natural Law and are denying those that they wish to murder, their Right to Life. Under UK Law one has the right to protection against a potential murderer by the use of reasonable force.

Reasonable force is always proportional to the threat presented at the time and must never exceed this, lest it be termed 'excessive force'. There is no specific definition of what does or does not constitute reasonable force. This is because UK lawmakers understand that each situation is different.

Since reasonable force is permitted under UK law to prevent yourself being murdered (presumably this is true in many other countries), then such reasonable force may be used by persons under attack from the pharmaceutical industry and their "Covid19" "vaccines" strategies. The advice given in Chapter 17 would be considered to fall well within the UK law requirements on reasonableness.

CHAPTER 21

TOWARDS A BETTER FUTURE

New 'Alliances' are Forming All Over The World

'World Doctors Alliance'

'Doctors for Information' and 'Doctors for Truth' have joined forces with similar groups of practitioners around the world in the **'World Doctors Alliance'**

This historic alliance connects more than one hundred thousand medical professionals around the world. **They reveal how the "pandemic" is the greatest crime in history and offer solid scientific evidence for this claim.** ***They also take legal actions against governments who are playing along with this criminal operation.***

Ref: https://worlddoctorsalliance.com/

Ref: https://stopworldcontrol.com/proof/

'World Freedom Alliance'

Similarly, the World Freedom Alliance was formed - a network of attorneys, medical experts, politicians, bankers, and many other professionals who are working together to expose the 'Covid Crime', and who are starting to build a new world of freedom. ***They want to make sure these kinds of worldwide scams that destroy millions of lives can never occur again.***

https://worldfreedomalliance.org/

'Hardwick Alliance'

The Hardwick Alliance for Real Ecology (HARE)

'Holistic in outlook, pragmatic in action'

'HARE' was formed in February 2020 at Hardwick House, Whitchurch-on-Thames in Oxfordshire, UK with the task of creating a united and purposeful front to expose, challenge and reverse our present deeply oppressive, corrupted and degraded political and economic systems.

Ref: https://hardwickalliance.org/

'The No Corruption Alliance' - based in UK

Join the revolution! The No Corruption Alliance is an independent alliance to replace the system with completely independent MPs. It is a fresh approach to the current corrupt system. We are compiling a directory of candidates who have all signed our pledge to prevent corruption. We are providing the tools to vet these candidates so everyone can feel satisfied in their integrity.

Ref: www.nocorruptionalliance.com

The four Global Alliances above, have come into being since the outbreak of "Covid19" as people have become aware, to varying degrees, of the global evil and murder that has taken place under the cloak of "health care", and that this evil and murder appear to be approved of by their "elected" "representatives" or at the very least, the "elected" "representatives" are docile, compliant, intellectually moribund zombies.

These Global Alliances are Steps in the Right Direction

The "elite", powerful, wealthy few, have ruled over the impoverished many since the beginning of 'civilisation': the Romans, Persians, Greeks, Egyptians etc. However, this form of regime became the most thoroughly institutional in European Feudalism – 9th to 15th centuries which may be considered to be the first form of capitalism. This was followed by further forms of capitalism: mercantilism, industrial capitalism, post-industrial capitalism (information/data technology) to **the current insanity of Harari and Schwab's 'Unelected Globalist Supra Sovereign State Surveillance Digital Transhumanism Capitalism'**

i.e. **'UGSS-SSDTC'**

Ref: 'Save Yourself Save Us All' Chapter 1.

Ref: https://saveyourselfsaveusall.co.uk/

The reader may wonder if the double **'SS'** is a reference to Hitler's SS. Rest assured it must be pure coincidence!

This global "elite" have now made a huge historical mistake. They have drawn up a preposterous "plan" that is contrary to Natural Law. As explained in Chapter 20, all Life or Beings of any manner whatsoever, that comes into being, (becoming a form of life) - through Natural means, by definition must have a right to the continuance of that life or being. This is inherent in Natural Law.

What we are observing in the case of this "Covid19" "vaccines" business, is that the Truth of Natural Law is being violated by some very low intelligence and very low sense of Ethics and Morals but powerful, rich, and dangerous people. The problem with these people is that, apart from their lack of Ethics and Morals they have a psychological profile, over which they have little or no control, which does not permit them to be otherwise. Any plan that violates Natural Law will fail. The Maoist Plan failed, the Stalinist Plan failed, Hitler's plan failed. They all failed because they violated Natural Law which necessitates *a priori* the furtherance of all Natural Life. These "plans" all failed because they did not permit the furtherance of all Natural Life, specifically in this case - Human Life. They restricted it and killed it without limit, without remorse, without giving a damn! So, to with **the current insanity of Harari and Schwab's 'Unelected Globalist Supra Sovereign State Surveillance Digital Transhumanism Capitalism'.**

i.e. **'UGSS-SSDTC'**

Already, the truth of what these evil people are doing along with say 300 to 1,000 others, is well known the world over by intelligent and powerful people as these words are being written in November 2022. Indeed, it has been well known for a long time. Quietly and steadily these agents for TRUTH are working to stop this madness. It is not fair to give all the "Satanic" glory to Harari and Schwab. These are merely greedy, stupid, 'front-it' glove- puppets, as are Bill Gates, Dr Fauci, George Soros, Ursula Gertrud von der Leyen, the Rockefellers, the Rothschilds, Big Pharma, Big Tech etc. The real power behind this idiocy lies with those who rarely show themselves, but they are well known to those who are interested enough to seek them.

These people have over-reached themselves with a poorly thought out and even more poorly executed "plan". They have been FOUND OUT!

For their plan to work they needed 90% to 95% of the world "vaccinated" with their poisons and for the "vaccinated" persons data to be held digitally and available globally to the "elite". See 'Great Reset Danger' diagram on page viii, page 55. However only 62.4% of the global population have received one "vaccination" to the current date of 24th November 2022.

Ref:https://ourworldindata.org/covid-vaccinations#what-share-of-the-population-has-received-at-least-one-dose-of-vaccine

Since the "elite" have failed and they are being exposed more and more on a daily basis, then no matter how long they resist, they will eventually fall. The level of corruption at such a high, global, pan sovereignty level and with such enormity of purpose to do evil is so great that the only way to resolve this crisis is by rooting this corruption out from the very top to the very bottom. This is not the first time that a civilisation has crumbled owing to corruption which tends to creep into a system whereby the 'fat cats' have got too fat and become complacent. All empires crumble into dust in this way: Egyptian, Greek, Roman etc.

The Opportunity for Change

What the above scenario offers the many of the world, is a root and branch opportunity for long lasting change for the better. Not only the opportunity to rid the world of the evil "elite" Evil300 but to restructure global society throughout.

It has been shown, quite clearly, that GGDP - Growth of Gross Domestic Product on a nationalistic competitive continuum platform was a dead paradigm before it really got started.

Eternal, perpetual, increase in GDP on a quarterly, on quarterly, on quarterly, on quarterly (yawn) basis (the font of all Capitalist "Wisdom") was never anything other than a completely moronic idea.

Ref: 'Save Yourself Save Us All' https://saveyourselfsaveusall.co.uk/

Jack Welch, CEO General Electric USA, the greatest Global Corporate CEO of the last century stated:

"On the face of it, shareholder value is the dumbest idea in the world,"

The world needs to look at an evolutionary, though radical new structure, once we have cleaned out the vermin and all that remains of them.

A New Global Strategy - In Summary:

1. Rid the world of these Unelected Evil Totalitarian Globalists, (Evil300) bring those responsible to justice
2. Break up Big Pharma and bring those responsible to justice
3. Move towards holistic, natural health treatments
4. Bring in population control by pragmatic legislation
5. Forget GDP as a paradigm, it's long dead
6. Re-identify the Role of Sovereign Governments – what use are these people who 'represent' us and what do we need from them
7. Minimise the role of Sovereign Governments
8. Maximise the role of the individual, family, and local community
9. Have all sovereign governments legislate that there **must never** be a cross-over between AI/Robotics/Machine Learning, and the Human Brain and or Nervous System. There must be an 'ocean of thick blood' that separates them to eternity
10. Ensure that the legislature and judiciary is thoroughly independent of the executive
11. Instigate tests of proficiency and ethics for Government elected representatives
12. Any revelations of corruption and the elected representative is immediately dismissed from post
13. Outlaw any financial benefit from Government office on leaving office for a minimum of 10 years. Achieving public service cabinet office or other as a route to earning vast sums of money after leaving (or being sacked) from that office is not a gravy train career path to be encouraged. The most hideous recent example is Tony Blair "man" of war crimes – Kofi Annan, Secretary General United Nations.
14. Move towards local communities governing local areas with a minimum sized sovereign government in public/private partnership cooperation providing a minimum national infrastructure i.e., roads, power
15. Create global alliances as shown above to integrate with 17. below
16. Create community alliances that will replace the corrupt systems of City and Town Councils
17. Instigate a culture where VIRTUE is 'king'

18. Reward the individual based on their VIRTUE contribution to the local community
19. True long-term happiness to be sought through true self-realisation not through acquisitive greed driven, material "wealth"
20. Overcome and dispel your fear and greed
21. BE HAPPY in each and every day of your Journey

"To finish the moment, to find the journey's end in every step of the road, to live the greatest number of good hours, is wisdom." - Ralph Waldo Emerson 1803 – 1882

APPENDIX I

Introduction only – APPENDIX I is a Free Download PDF File on Website: https://covid19compensation2022.com/

Letter and Report that is included in this book sent to Baroness Hallett UK Covid-19 Public Inquiry, House of Lords, London. Latest Letter and Report sent on 12th October 2022, previous similar copies sent on 23rd June 2022 and 2nd August 2022 – the two more recent letters/reports were made under the UK Freedom of Information Act 2000 FOIA. There have been NO replies. This is unlawful. The UK Freedom of Information Act 2000 clearly states that replies from Government and Public Authorities to FOIA requests must be made within 20 working days of receipt of the request.

Latest Letter, Report, Report Appendices to:

Recipients	**Office at the Time of Covid 2019-2022-**
Boris Johnson	**Prime Minister**
Matt Hancock	**Health & Social Care**
Nadhim Zahawi	**"Covid" ""Vaccine" Deployment**
Michael Gove	**Cabinet Office**
Sajid Javid	**Health & Social Care**
Suella Braverman	**Attorney General**
Priti Patel	**Home Office**
Baroness Hallett	**Chair Covid Inquiry 2012-**
Independent Covid Inquiry 2012-	**House of Lords Inquiry**
Christopher Whitty	**Chief Medical Officer/Chief Medical Advisor**
Patrick Vallance	**Chief Scientific Advisor**
June Munro Raine	**CEO MHRA** – Medicines & Healthcare Products Regulatory Agency
Charlie Massey	**CEO GMC** – General Medical Council
Amanda Pritchard	**CEO NHS** – National Health Service
Neil Ferguson	**Researcher** – Imperial College, London
John Witherow	**'The Times'**
Chris Evans	**'The Telegraph'**
Ian Hislop	**'Private Eye'**

APPENDIX II

Freedom of Information Request for Proof of Existence of "Sars-Cov2" and that the "Vaccines" do not contain harmful Graphene Oxide or other poisons placed upon General Medical Council GMC and UK NHS and their replies. The replies from GMC, NHS and Nadhim Zahawi were sent to the Editor when initiated by other correspondence by email. There were NO replies to this particular piece of correspondence.

Professor Ian Abbs
Chief Executive
St Thomas' Hospital
Vaccination Centre 1
Westminster Bridge Road
London SE1 7EH

15th October 2022

COVID19 VACCINATION

FREEDOM OF INFORMATION ACT 2000 FOI REQUEST

Thank you for your offer to vaccinate me against Covid19. Before I proceed to accept your offer of Covid19 vaccination, I would like to ensure that I am able to provide you with **my informed consent.**

Please provide:

1. Proof of the existence of the SARS-CoV-2 virus by research describing the isolation of the SARS-CoV-2 virus aka COVID-19 in human beings, by scientific analysis of samples taken directly from a diseased patient, where the patient samples were not first combined with any other source of genetic material. Note: The word "isolate" means: a thing (SARS-CoV-2/COVID-19) is separated from all other material surrounding it. I am not requesting information where so-called "isolation" of SARS-CoV-2 refers to: - the culturing of something, or - the performance of an amplification test (PCR), or - the sequencing of something. The research study methodology may require the use of Koch Postulates.
2. Proof that all the vaccines approved for use in UK such as: Moderna vaccine, Oxford/AstraZeneca vaccine, Pfizer/BioNTech vaccine and any other vaccine approved for use in UK but not here listed, are all safe for human use and do not contain any graphene oxide or any other substances in any way harmful to humans.

Note that if this material requested in points 1. and 2. above is not readily available to your organization then it should be readily available from one or more of the persons on the list overleaf. This Notice under the Freedom of Information Act 2000 is simultaneously served on the list of persons overleaf by Royal Mail. All recipients are formally requested to reply individually, being independently causal agents in this matter of SARS-CoV-2/COVID-19.

Recipient List	**Office** (at the time of Covid19 – 2019/2020 onwards)
Boris Johnson	**Prime Minister**
Matt Hancock	**Health & Social Care**
Nadhim Zahawi	**"Covid" "Vaccine" Deployment**
Michael Gove	**Cabinet Office**
Sajid Javid	**Health & Social Care**
Suella Braverman	**Attorney General**
Priti Patel	**Home Office**
Baroness Hallett	**Chair Covid Inquiry 2021-**
Christopher Whitty	**Chief Medical Officer/Chief Medical Advisor**
Patrick Vallance	**Chief Scientific Advisor**
June Munro Raine	**CEO MHRA** - Medicines and Healthcare Products Regulatory Agency
Charlie Massey	**CEO GMC** – General Medical Council
Amanda Pritchard	**CEO NHS** – National Health Service
Neil Ferguson	**Researcher** - Imperial College, London
Dr Gillian Ostrowski	**Medical Doctor** formerly NHS Bridge Lane Practice/South West London Covid19 Testing Centre – This FOI Request is made under this former employment
Dr Johannes Coetzee	**Medical Doctor** NHS Bridge Lane Practice
Joanne Lawson	**Practice Management** NHS Bridge Lane Practice

Your reply by email with attachments or URL links to the material requested will suffice.

END OF LETTER

REPLIES RECEIVED

UK General Medical Council GMC
reply: NO RECORD [available relating to this FOIA 2000 request]
dated: 6th December 2022

UK National Health Service NHS
reply: NO RECORD [available relating to this FOIA 2000 request]
dated: 25th November 2022

Nadhim Zahawi "Covid" "Vaccine" Deployment
reply: NO RECORD [available relating to this FOIA 2000 request]
dated: 13th January 2023

APPENDIX III

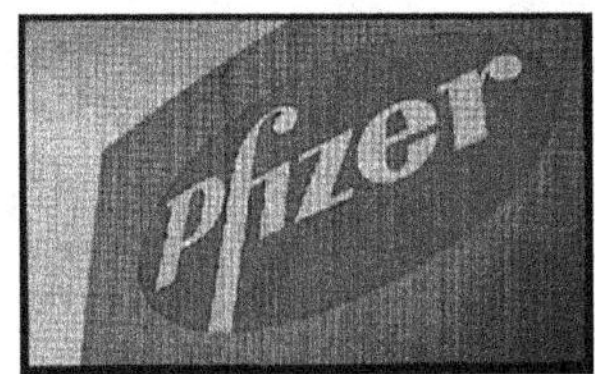

PFIZER

Official Report Appendix 1.

5.3.6 CUMULATIVE ANALYSIS OF POST-AUTHORIZATION <u>ADVERSE EVENT REPORTS</u> OF PF-07302048 (BNT162B2) RECEIVED THROUGH 28-FEB-2021

Pfizer/BioNTech's proposal for the clinical and post-authorization safety data package for the Biologics License Application (BLA) for our investigational COVID-19 Vaccine (BNT162b2)

c. <u>10 pages, 2,291-word count</u>

<u>APPENDIX 1. LIST OF ["Covid19" "Vaccines"] ADVERSE EVENTS OF SPECIAL INTEREST</u>

1p36 deletion syndrome;2-Hydroxyglutaric aciduria;5'nucleotidase increased;Acoustic neuritis;Acquired C1 inhibitor deficiency;Acquired epidermolysis bullosa;Acquired epileptic aphasia;Acute cutaneous lupus erythematosus;Acute disseminated encephalomyelitis;Acute encephalitis with refractory, repetitive partial seizures;Acute febrile neutrophilic dermatosis;Acute flaccid myelitis;Acute haemorrhagic leukoencephalitis;Acute haemorrhagic oedema of infancy;Acute kidney injury;Acute macular outer retinopathy;Acute motor axonal neuropathy;Acute motor-sensory axonal neuropathy;Acute myocardial infarction;Acute respiratory distress syndrome;Acute respiratory failure;Addison's disease;Administration site thrombosis;Administration site vasculitis;Adrenal thrombosis;Adverse event following immun isation;Ageusia;Agranulocytosis;Air embolism;Alanine aminotransferase abnormal;Alanine aminotransferase increased;Alcoholic seizure;Allergic bronchopulmonary mycosis;Allergic oedema;Alloimmune hepatitis;Alopecia areata;Alpers disease;Alveolar proteinosis;Ammonia abnormal;Ammonia increased;Amniotic cavity infection;Amygdalohippocampectomy;Amyl oid arthropathy;Amyloidosis;Amyloidosis senile;Anaphylactic reaction;Anaphylactic shock;Anaphylactic transfusion reaction;Anaphylactoid reaction;Anaphylactoid shock;Anaphylactoid syndrome of pregnancy;Angioedema;Angiopathic neuropathy;Ankylosing spondylitis;Anosmia;Antiacetylcholine receptor antibody positive;Anti-actin antibody positive;Anti-aquaporin-4 antibody positive;Anti-basal ganglia antibody positive;Anti-cyclic citrullinated peptide antibody positive;Anti-epithelial antibody positive;Anti-erythrocyte antibody positive;Anti-exosome complex antibody positive;AntiGAD antibody negative;Anti-GAD antibody positive;Anti-ganglioside antibody positive;Antigliadin antibody positive;Anti-glomerular basement membrane antibody positive;Anti-glomerular basement membrane disease;Anti-glycyl-tRNA synthetase antibody positive;Anti-HLA antibody test positive;Anti-IA2 antibody positive;Anti-insulin antibody increased;Anti-insulin antibody positive;Anti-insulin receptor antibody increased;Antiinsulin receptor antibody positive;Anti-interferon antibody negative;Anti-interferon antibody positive;Anti-islet cell antibody positive;Antimitochondrial antibody positive;Anti-muscle specific kinase antibody positive;Anti-myelin-associated glycoprotein antibodies positive; Anti-myelin-associated glycoprotein associated polyneuropathy;Antimyocardial antibody positive;Anti-neuronal antibody positive;Antineutrophil cytoplasmic antibody increased;Antineutrophil cytoplasmic antibody positive;Anti-neutrophil cytoplasmic antibody positive vasculitis;Anti-NMDA antibody positive;Antinuclear antibody increased;Antinuclear antibody positive;Antiphospholipid antibodies positive;Antiphospholipid syndrome; Anti-platelet antibody positive;Anti-prothrombin antibody positive;Antiribosomal P antibody positive;Anti-RNA polymerase III antibody positive;Anti-saccharomyces cerevisiae antibody test positive;Anti-sperm antibody positive;Anti-SRP antibody positive;Antisynthetase syndrome;Anti-thyroid antibody positive;Anti-transglutaminase antibody increased;Anti-VGCC antibody positive;AntiVGKC antibody positive; Anti-vimentin antibody positive;Antiviral prophylaxis;Antiviral treatment;Anti-zinc transporter 8 antibody positive;Aortic embolus;Aortic thrombosis;Aortitis;Aplasia pure red cell;Aplastic anaemia;Application site thrombosis;Application site vasculitis;Arrhythmia;Arterial bypass occlusion;Arterial bypass thrombosis;Arterial thrombosis;Arteriovenous fistula thrombosis;Arteriovenous graft site stenosis; Arteriovenous graft thrombosis;Arteritis;Arteritis 090177e196ea1800\Approved\ Approved On: 30-A pr-2021 09:26 (GMT) FDA-CBER-2021-5683-0000083 BNT162b2 5.3.6 Cumulative Analysis of Post-authorization Adverse Event Reports CONFIDENTIAL coronary;Arthralgia;Arthritis;Arthritis enteropathic;Ascites;Aseptic cavernous sinus thrombosis;Aspartate aminotransferase abnormal;Aspartate aminotransferase increased;Aspartate-glutamate-transporter deficiency;AST to platelet ratio index increased;AST/ALT ratio abnormal;Asthma;Asymptomatic COVID19;Ataxia;Atheroembolis m;Atonic seizures;Atrial thrombosis;Atrophic thyroiditis;Atypical benign partial epilepsy;Atypical pneumonia;Aura;Autoantibody positive;Autoimmune anaemia;Autoimmune aplastic anaemia;Autoimmune arthritis;Autoimmune blistering disease;Autoimmune cholangitis;Autoimmune colitis;Autoimmune demyelinating disease;Autoimmune dermatitis;Autoimmune disorder;Autoimmune encephalopathy;Autoimmune endocrine disorder;Autoimmune enteropathy;Autoimmune eye disorder;Autoimmune haemolytic anaemia;Autoimmune heparin-induced thrombocytopenia;Autoimmune hepatitis;Autoimmune hyperlipidaemia;Autoimmune hypothyroidism;Autoimmune inner ear disease;Autoimmune lung disease;Autoimmune lymphoproliferative syndrome;Autoimmune myocarditis;Autoimmune myositis;Autoimmune nephritis;Autoimmune neuropathy;Autoimmune neutropenia;Autoimmune pancreatitis;Autoimmune pancytopenia;Autoimmune pericarditis;Autoimmune retinopathy;Autoimmune thyroid disorder;Autoimmune thyroiditis;Autoimmune uveitis;Autoinflammation with infantile enterocolitis;Autoinflammatory disease;Automatism epileptic;Autonomic nervous system imbalance;Autonomic seizure;Axial spondyloarthritis;Axillary vein thrombosis;Axonal and demyelinating polyneuropathy;Axonal neuropathy;Bacterascites;Baltic myoclonic epilepsy;Band sensation;Basedow's disease;Basilar artery thrombosis;Basophilopenia;B-cell aplasia;Behcet's syndrome;Benign ethnic neutropenia;Benign familial neonatal convulsions;Benign familial pemphigus;Benign rolandic epilepsy;Beta-2 glycoprotein antibody positive;Bickerstaff's encephalitis;Bile output abnormal;Bile output decreased;Biliary ascites;Bilirubin conjugated abnormal;Bilirubin conjugated increased;Bilirubin urine present;Biopsy liver abnormal;Biotinidase deficiency;Birdshot chorioretinopathy;Blood alkaline phosphatase abnormal;Blood alkaline phosphatase increased;Blood bilirubin abnormal;Blood bilirubin increased;Blood bilirubin unconjugated increased;Blood cholinesterase abnormal;Blood cholinesterase decreased;Blood pressure decreased;Blood pressure diastolic decreased;Blood pressure systolic decreased; Blue toe syndrome;Brachiocephalic vein thrombosis;Brain stem embolism;Brain stem thrombosis;Bromosulphthalein test abnormal;Bronchial oedema;Bronchitis;Bronchitis mycoplasmal;Bronchitis viral;Bronchopulmonary aspergillosis allergic;Bronchospasm;BuddC hiari syndrome;Bulbar palsy;Butterfly rash;C1q nephropathy;Caesarean section;Calcium embolism;Capillaritis;Caplan's syndrome;Cardiac amyloidosis;Cardiac arrest;Cardiac failure;Cardiac failure acute;Cardiac sarcoidosis;Cardiac ventricular thrombosis;Cardiogenic shock;Cardiolipin antibody positive;Cardiopulmonary failure;Cardio-respiratory arrest;Cardio-respiratory distress;Cardiovascular insufficiency;Carotid arterial embolus;Carotid artery thrombosis;Cataplexy;Catheter site thrombosis;Catheter site vasculitis;Cavernous sinus thrombosis;CDKL5 deficiency disorder;CEC syndrome;Cement embolism;Central nervous system lupus;Central nervous system vasculitis;Cerebellar artery thrombosis;Cerebellar embolism;Cerebral amyloid angiopathy;Cerebral arteritis;Cerebral artery embolism; Cerebral artery thrombosis;Cerebral gas embolism;Cerebral microembolism;Cerebral septic infarct;Cerebral thrombosis;Cerebral venous sinus thrombosis;Cerebral venous thrombosis;Cerebrospinal thrombotic 090177e196ea1800\Approved\Approved On: 30-A pr-2021 09:26 (GMT) FDA-CBER-2021-5683-0000084 BNT162b2 5.3.6 Cumulative Analysis of Post-authorization Adverse Event Reports CONFIDENTIAL tamponade;Cerebrovascular accident;Change in seizure presentation;Chest discomfort;ChildPugh-Turcotte score abnormal;Child-Pugh-Turcotte score increased; Chillblains;Choking;Choking sensation;Cholangitis sclerosing;Chronic autoimmune glomerulonephritis;Chronic cutaneous lupus erythematosus;Chronic fatigue syndrome;Chronic gastritis;Chronic inflammatory demyelinating polyradiculoneuropathy;Chronic lymphocytic inflammation with pontine perivascular enhancement responsive to steroids;Chronic recurrent multifocal osteomyelitis;Chronic respiratory failure;Chronic spontaneous urticaria;Circulatory collapse;Circumoral oedema;Circumoral swelling;Clinically isolated syndrome;Clonic convulsion;Coeliac disease;Cogan's syndrome;Cold agglutinins positive;Cold type haemolytic anaemia;Colitis;Colitis erosive;Colitis herpes;Colitis microscopic;Colitis ulcerative;Collagen disorder;Collagen-vascular disease;Complement factor abnormal;Complement factor C1 decreased;Complement factor C2 decreased;Complement factor C3 decreased;Complement factor C4 decreased;Complement factor decreased;Computerised tomogram liver abnormal;Concentric sclerosis;Congenital anomaly;Congenital bilateral perisylvian syndrome;Congenital herpes simplex infection;Congenital myasthenic syndrome;Congenital varicella infection;Congestive hepatopathy;Convulsion in childhood;Convulsions local;Convulsive threshold lowered;Coombs positive haemolytic anaemia;Coronary artery disease;Coronary artery embolism;Coronary artery thrombosis;Coronary bypass thrombosis;Coronavirus infection;Coronavirus test;Coronavirus test negative;Coronavirus test positive;Corpus callosotomy;Cough;Cough variant asthma;COVID-19;COVID-19 immunisation;COVID-19 pneumonia;COVID-19 prophylaxis;COVID-19 treatment;Cranial nerve disorder;Cranial nerve palsies multiple;Cranial nerve paralysis;CREST syndrome;Crohn's disease;Cryofibrinogenaemia;Cryoglobulinaemia;CSF oligoclonal band present;CSWS syndrome;Cutaneous amyloidosis;Cutaneous lupus erythematosus;Cutaneous sarcoidosis;Cutaneous vasculitis;Cyanosis;Cyclic neutropenia;Cystitis interstitial;Cytokine release syndrome;Cytokine storm;De novo purine synthesis inhibitors associated acute inflammatory syndrome;Death neonatal;Deep vein thrombosis;Deep vein thrombosis postoperative;Deficiency of bile secretion;Deja vu;Demyelinating polyneuropathy;Demyelinat ion;Dermatitis;Dermatitis bullous;Dermatitis herpetiformis;Dermatomyositis;Device embolisation;Device related thrombosis;Diabetes mellitus;Diabetic ketoacidosis;Diabetic mastopathy;Dialysis amyloidosis;Dialysis membrane reaction;Diastolic hypotension;Diffuse vasculitis;Digital pitting scar;Disseminated intravascular coagulation;Disseminated intravascular coagulation in newborn;Disseminated neonatal herpes simplex;Disseminated varicella;Disseminated varicella zoster vaccine virus infection;Disseminated varicella zoster virus infection;DNA antibody positive;Double cortex syndrome;Double stranded DNA antibody positive;Dreamy state;Dressler's syndrome;Drop attacks;Drug withdrawal convulsions;Dyspnoea;Early infantile epileptic encephalopathy with burst-suppression;Eclampsia;Eczema herpeticum;Embolia cutis medicamentosa;Embolic cerebellar infarction;Embolic cerebral infarction;Embolic pneumonia;Embolic stroke;Embolism;Embolism arterial;Embolism venous;Encephalitis;Encephalitis allergic;Encephalitis autoimmune;Encephalitis brain stem;Encephalitis haemorrhagic;Encephalitis periaxialis diffusa;Encephalitis post immunisation; Encephalomyelitis;Encephalopathy;Endocrine disorder;Endocrine ophthalmopathy; Endotracheal intubation;Enteritis;Enteritis leukopenic;Enterobacter pneumonia;Enterocolitis;E nteropathic spondylitis;Eosinopenia;Eosinophilic 090177e196ea1800\Approved\Approved On: 30-A pr-2021 09:26 (GMT) FDA-CBER-2021-5683-0000085 BNT162b2 5.3.6 Cumulative Analysis of Post-authorization Adverse Event Reports CONFIDENTIAL fasciitis;Eosinophilic granulomatosis with polyangiitis;Eosinophilic oesophagitis;Epidermolys is;Epilepsy;Epilepsy surgery;Epilepsy with myoclonic-atonic seizures;Epileptic aura;Epileptic psychosis;Erythema;Erythema induratum;Erythema multiforme;Erythema nodosum;Evans syndrome;Exanthema subitum;Expanded disability status scale score decreased;Expanded disability status scale score increased;Exposure to communicable disease;Exposure to SARS-CoV-2;Eye oedema;Eye pruritus;Eye swelling;Eyelid oedema;Face oedema; Facial paralysis;Facial paresis;Faciobrachial dystonic seizure;Fat embolism;Febrile convulsion;Febrile infection-related epilepsy syndrome;Febrile neutropenia;Felty's syndrome;Femoral artery embolism;Fibrillary glomerulonephritis;Fibromyalgia;Flushing;Foa ming at mouth;Focal cortical resection;Focal dyscognitive seizures;Foetal distress syndrome;Foetal placental thrombosis;Foetor hepaticus;Foreign body embolism; Frontal lobe epilepsy;Fulminant type 1 diabetes mellitus;Galactose elimination capacity test abnormal;Galactose elimination capacity test decreased;Gamma-glutamyltransferase abnormal;Gamma-glutamyltransferase increased;Gastritis herpes;Gastrointestinal amyloidosis;Gelastic seizure;Generalised onset non-motor seizure;Generalised tonic-clonic seizure;Genital herpes;Genital herpes simplex;Genital herpes zoster;Giant cell arteritis;Glomerulonephritis;Glomerulonephritis membranoproliferative;Glomerulonephritis membranous;Glomerulonephritis rapidly progressive;Glossopharyngeal nerve paralysis;Glucose transporter type 1 deficiency syndrome;Glutamate dehydrogenase increased;Glycocholic acid increased;GM2 gangliosidosis;Goodpasture's syndrome; Graft thrombosis;Granulocytopenia;Granulocytopenia neonatal;Granulomatosis with polyangiitis;Granulomatous dermatitis;Grey matter heterotopia;Guanase increased;GuillainBarre syndrome;Haemolytic anaemia;Haemophagocytic lymphohistiocytosis;Haemorrhage;Haemorrhagic ascites;Haemorrhagic disorder; Haemorrhagic pneumonia;Haemorrhagic varicella syndrome;Haemorrhagic vasculitis;Hantavirus pulmonary infection;Hashimoto's encephalopathy;Hashitoxicosis; Hemimegalencephaly;Henoch-Schonlein purpura;HenochSchonlein purpura nephritis; Hepaplastin abnormal;Hepaplastin decreased;Heparin-induced thrombocytopenia;Hepatic amyloidosis;Hepatic artery embolism;Hepatic artery flow decreased;Hepatic artery thrombosis;Hepatic enzyme abnormal;Hepatic enzyme decreased;Hepatic enzyme increased;Hepatic fibrosis marker abnormal;Hepatic fibrosis marker increased;Hepatic function abnormal;Hepatic hydrothorax;Hepatic hypertrophy;Hepatic hypoperfusion;Hepatic lymphocytic infiltration;Hepatic mass;Hepatic pain;Hepatic sequestration;Hepatic vascular resistance increased;Hepatic vascular thrombosis;Hepatic vein embolism;Hepatic vein thrombosis;Hepatic venous pressure gradient abnormal;Hepatic venous pressure gradient incre ased;Hepatitis;Hepatobiliary scan abnormal;Hepatomegaly;Hepatosplenomegaly;Hereditary angioedema with C1 esterase inhibitor deficiency;Herpes dermatitis;Herpes gestationis;Herpes oesophagitis;Herpes ophthalmic;Herpes pharyngitis;Herpes sepsis;Herpes simplex; Herpes simplex cervicitis;Herpes simplex colitis;Herpes simplex encephalitis;Herpes simplex gastritis;Herpes simplex hepatitis;Herpes simplex meningitis;Herpes simplex meningoencephalitis;Herpes simplex meningomyelitis;Herpes simplex necrotising retinopathy;Herpes simplex oesophagitis;Herpes simplex otitis externa;Herpes simplex pharyngitis;Herpes simplex pneumonia;Herpes simplex reactivation;Herpes simplex sepsis;Herpes simplex viraemia;Herpes simplex virus conjunctivitis neonatal;Herpes simplex visceral;Herpes virus 090177e196ea1800\Approved\Approved On: 30-A pr-2021 09:26 (GMT) FDA-CBER-2021-5683-0000086 BNT162b2 5.3.6 Cumulative Analysis of Post-authorization Adverse Event Reports CONFIDENTIAL infection;Herpes zoster; Herpes zoster cutaneous disseminated;Herpes zoster infection neurological;Herpes zoster meningitis;Herpes zoster meningoencephalitis;Herpes zoster meningomyelitis;Herpes zoster meningoradiculitis;Herpes zoster necrotising retinopathy;Herpes zoster oticus;Herpes zoster pharyngitis;Herpes zoster reactivation;Herpetic radiculopathy;Histone antibody positive;Hoigne's syndrome;Human herpesvirus 6 encephalitis;Human herpesvirus 6 infection;Human herpesvirus 6 infection reactivation;Human herpesvirus 7 infection;Human herpesvirus 8 infection;Hyperammonaemia;Hyperbilirubinaemia;Hypercholia;

Hypergammaglobulinaemia benign monoclonal;Hyperglycaemic seizure;Hypersensitivity; Hypersensitivity vasculitis;Hyperthyroidism;Hypertransaminasaemia;Hyperventilation; Hypoalbuminaemia;H ypocalcaemic seizure;Hypogammaglobulinaemia;Hypoglossal nerve paralysis;Hypoglossal nerve paresis;Hypoglycaemic seizure;Hyponatraemic seizure;Hypotension;Hypotensive crisis;Hypothenar hammer syndrome;Hypothyroidism; Hypoxia;Idiopathic CD4 lymphocytopenia;Idiopathic generalised epilepsy;Idiopathic interstitial pneumonia;Idiopathic neutropenia;Idiopathic pulmonary fibrosis;IgA nephropathy;IgM nephropathy;IIIrd nerve paralysis;IIIrd nerve paresis;Iliac artery embolism;Immune thrombocytopenia;Immunemediated adverse reaction;Immune-mediated cholangitis;Immune-mediated cholestasis;Immune-mediated cytopenia; Immune-mediated encephalitis;Immune-mediated encephalopathy;Immune-mediated endocrinopathy;Immune-mediated enterocolitis;Immunemediated gastritis;Immune-mediated hepatic disorder;Immune-mediated hepatitis;Immunemediated hyperthyroidism; Immune-mediated hypothyroidism;Immune-mediated myocarditis;Immune-mediated myositis;Immune-mediated nephritis;Immune-mediated neuropathy;Immune-mediated pancreatitis;Immune-mediated pneumonitis;Immune-mediated renal disorder;Immune-mediated thyroiditis;Immune-mediated uveitis;Immunoglobulin G4 related disease;Immunoglobulins abnormal;Implant site thrombosis;Inclusion body myositis; Infantile genetic agranulocytosis;Infantile spasms;Infected vasculitis;Infective thrombosis; Inflammation;Inflammatory bowel disease;Infusion site thrombosis;Infusion site vasculitis;Injection site thrombosis;Injection site urticaria;Injection site vasculitis;Instillation site thrombosis;Insulin autoimmune syndrome;Interstitial granulomatous dermatitis; Interstitial lung disease;Intracardiac mass;Intracardiac thrombus;Intracranial pressure increased;Intrapericardial thrombosis;Intrinsic factor antibody abnormal;Intrinsic factor antibody positive;IPEX syndrome;Irregular breathing;IRVAN syndrome;IVth nerve paralysis;IVth nerve paresis;JC polyomavirus test positive;JC virus CSF test positive; Jeavons syndrome;Jugular vein embolism;Jugular vein thrombosis;Juvenile idiopathic arthritis;Juvenile myoclonic epilepsy;Juvenile polymyositis;Juvenile psoriatic arthritis; Juvenile spondyloarthritis;Kaposi sarcoma inflammatory cytokine syndrome;Kawasaki's disease;Kayser-Fleischer ring;Keratoderma blenorrhagica;Ketosisprone diabetes mellitus;Kounis syndrome;Lafora's myoclonic epilepsy;Lambl's excrescences;Laryngeal dyspnoea;Laryngeal oedema;Laryngeal rheumatoid arthritis;Laryngospasm;Laryngotracheal oedema;Latent autoimmune diabetes in adults;LE cells present;Lemierre syndrome;Lennox-Gastaut syndrome;Leucine aminopeptidase increased;Leukoencephalomyelitis;Leukoencephal opathy;Leukopenia;Leukopenia neonatal;Lewis-Sumner syndrome;Lhermitte's sign;Lichen planopilaris;Lichen planus;Lichen sclerosus;Limbic encephalitis;Linear IgA disease;Lip oedema;Lip swelling;Liver function test abnormal;Liver function test decreased;Liver function test increased;Liver induration;Liver injury;Liver iron concentration abnormal;Liver iron concentration 090177e196ea1800\Approved\Approved On: 30-A pr-2021 09:26 (GMT) FDA-CBER-2021-5683-0000087 BNT162b2 5.3.6 Cumulative Analysis of Post-authorization Adverse Event Reports CONFIDENTIAL increased;Liver opacity;Liver palpable;Liver sarcoidosis;Liver scan abnormal;Liver tenderness;Low birth weight baby;Lower respiratory tract herpes infection;Lower respiratory tract infection;Lower respiratory tract infection viral;Lung abscess;Lupoid hepatic cirrhosis;Lupus cystitis;Lupus encephalitis;Lupus endocarditis;Lupus enteritis;Lupus hepatitis;Lupus myocarditis;Lupus myositis;

Lupus nephritis;Lupus pancreatitis;Lupus pleurisy;Lupus pneumonitis;Lupus vasculitis; Lupus-like syndrome;Lymphocytic hypophysitis;Lymphocytopenia neonatal;Lymphopenia; MAGIC syndrome;Magnetic resonance imaging liver abnormal;Magnetic resonance proton density fat fraction measurement;Mahler sign;Manufacturing laboratory analytical testing issue;Manufacturing materials issue;Manufacturing production issue;Marburg's variant multiple sclerosis;Marchiafava-Bignami disease;Marine Lenhart syndrome;Mastocytic enterocolitis;Maternal exposure during pregnancy;Medical device site thrombosis; Medical device site vasculitis;MELAS syndrome;Meningitis;Meningitis aseptic;Meningitis herpes;Meningoencephalitis herpes simplex neonatal;Meningoencephalitis herpetic;Meningomyelitis herpes;MERS-CoV test;MERS-CoV test negative;MERS-CoV test positive;Mesangioproliferative glomerulonephritis;Mesenteric artery embolism;Mesenteric artery thrombosis;Mesenteric vein thrombosis;Metapneumovirus infection;Metastatic cutaneous Crohn's disease;Metastatic pulmonary embolism;Microangiopathy;Microembolism; Microscopic polyangiitis;Middle East respiratory syndrome;Migraine-triggered seizure;Miliary pneumonia;Miller Fisher syndrome;Mitochondrial aspartate aminotransferase increased;Mixed connective tissue disease;Model for end stage liver disease score abnormal;Model for end stage liver disease score increased;Molar ratio of total branched-chain amino acid to tyrosine;Molybdenum cofactor deficiency;Monocytopenia;Mononeuritis; Mononeuropathy multiplex;Morphoea;Morvan syndrome;Mouth swelling;Moyamoya disease;Multifocal motor neuropathy;Multiple organ dysfunction syndrome;Multiple sclerosis;Multiple sclerosis relapse;Multiple sclerosis relapse prophylaxis;Multiple subpial transection;Multisystem inflammatory syndrome in children;Muscular sarcoidosis; Myasthenia gravis;Myasthenia gravis crisis;Myasthenia gravis neonatal;Myasthenic syndrome;Myelitis;Myelitis transverse;Myocardial infarction;Myocarditis;Myocarditis post infection;Myoclonic epilepsy;Myoclonic epilepsy and ragged-red fibres;Myokymia;Myositis; Narcolepsy;Nasal herpes;Nasal obstruction;Necrotising herpetic retinopathy;Neonatal Crohn's disease;Neonatal epileptic seizure;Neonatal lupus erythematosus;Neonatal mucocutaneous herpes simplex;Neonatal pneumonia;Neonatal seizure;Nephritis;Nephrogenic systemic fibrosis;Neuralgic amyotrophy;Neuritis;Neuritis cranial;Neuromyelitis optica pseudo relapse;Neuromyelitis optica spectrum disorder;Neuromyotonia;Neuronal neuropathy;Neuropathy peripheral;Neuropathy, ataxia, retinitis pigmentosa syndrome;Neuropsychiatric lupus;Neurosarcoidosis;Neutropenia;Neutropenia neonatal;Neutropenic colitis;Neutropenic infection;Neutropenic sepsis;Nodular rash; Nodular vasculitis;Noninfectious myelitis;Noninfective encephalitis;Noninfective encephalomyelitis;Noninfective oophoritis;Obstetrical pulmonary embolism;Occupational exposure to communicable disease;Occupational exposure to SARS-CoV-2;Ocular hyperaemia;Ocular myasthenia;Ocular pemphigoid;Ocular sarcoidosis;Ocular vasculitis;Oculofacial paralysis;Oedema;Oedema blister;Oedema due to hepatic disease;Oedema mouth;Oesophageal achalasia;Ophthalmic artery thrombosis;Ophthalmic herpes simplex;Ophthalmic herpes zoster;Ophthalmic vein thrombosis;Optic neuritis;Optic 090177e196ea1800\Approved\Approved On: 30-A pr-2021 09:26 (GMT) FDA-CBER-2021-5683-0000088 BNT162b2 5.3.6 Cumulative Analysis of Post-authorization Adverse Event Reports CONFIDENTIAL neuropathy;Optic perineuritis;Oral herpes;Oral lichen planus;Oropharyngeal oedema;Oropharyngeal spasm;Oropharyngeal swelling;Osmotic demyelination syndrome;Ovarian vein thrombosis;Overlap syndrome;Paediatric autoimmune neuropsychiatric disorders associated with streptococcal infection;Paget-Schroetter syndrome;Palindromic rheumatism;Palisaded neutrophilic granulomatous dermatitis;Palmoplantar keratoderma;Palpable purpura;Pancreatitis;Panencephalitis; Papillophlebitis;Paracancerous pneumonia;Paradoxical embolism;Parainfluenzae viral laryngo tracheobronchitis;Paraneoplastic dermatomyositis;Paraneoplastic pemphigus;Paraneoplastic thrombosis;Paresis cranial nerve;Parietal cell antibody positive;Paroxysmal nocturnal haemoglobinuria;Partial seizures;Partial seizures with secondary generalisation;Patient isolation;Pelvic venous thrombosis;Pemphigoid;Pemphigus;Penile vein thrombosis;Pericarditi s;Pericarditis lupus;Perihepatic discomfort;Periorbital oedema;Periorbital swelling;Peripheral artery thrombosis;Peripheral embolism;Peripheral ischaemia;Peripheral vein thrombus extension;Periportal oedema;Peritoneal fluid protein abnormal;Peritoneal fluid protein decreased;Peritoneal fluid protein increased;Peritonitis lupus;Pernicious anaemia;Petit mal epilepsy;Pharyngeal oedema;Pharyngeal swelling;Pityriasis lichenoides et varioliformis acuta;Placenta praevia;Pleuroparenchymal fibroelastosis;Pneumobilia;Pneumonia; Pneumonia adenoviral;Pneumonia cytomegaloviral;Pneumonia herpes viral;Pneumonia influenzal;Pneumonia measles;Pneumonia mycoplasmal;Pneumonia necrotising;Pneumonia parainfluenzae viral;Pneumonia respiratory syncytial viral;Pneumonia viral;POEMS syndrome;Polyarteritis nodosa;Polyarthritis;Polychondritis;Polyglandular autoimmune syndrome type I;Polyglandular autoimmune syndrome type II;Polyglandular autoimmune syndrome type III;Polyglandular disorder;Polymicrogyria;Polymyalgia rheumatica;Polymyosit is;Polyneuropathy;Polyneuropathy idiopathic progressive;Portal pyaemia;Portal vein embolism;Portal vein flow decreased;Portal vein pressure increased;Portal vein thrombosis;Por tosplenomesenteric venous thrombosis;Post procedural hypotension;Post procedural pneumonia;Post procedural pulmonary embolism;Post stroke epilepsy;Post stroke seizure; Post thrombotic retinopathy;Post thrombotic syndrome;Post viral fatigue syndrome;Postictal headache;Postictal paralysis;Postictal psychosis;Postictal state;Postoperative respiratory distress;Postoperative respiratory failure;Postoperative thrombosis;Postpartum thrombosis;Postpartum venous thrombosis;Postpericardiotomy syndrome;Post-traumatic epilepsy;Postural orthostatic tachycardia syndrome;Precerebral artery thrombosis;Pre-eclampsia;Preictal state;Premature labour;Premature menopause;Primary amyloidosis;Primary biliary cholangitis;Primary progressive multiple sclerosis;Procedural shock;Proctitis herpes;Proctitis ulcerative;Product availability issue;Product distribution issue;Product supply issue;Progressive facial hemiatrophy;Progressive multifocal leukoencephalopathy; Progressive multiple sclerosis;Progressive relapsing multiple sclerosis;Prosthetic cardiac valve thrombosis;Pruritus;Pruritus allergic;Pseudovasculitis;Psoriasis;Psoriatic arthropathy;Pulmonary amyloidosis;Pulmonary artery thrombosis;Pulmonary embolism;Pulmonary fibrosis;Pulmonary haemorrhage;Pulmonary microemboli;Pulmonary oil microembolism;Pulmonary renal syndrome;Pulmonary sarcoidosis;Pulmonary sepsis;Pulmonary thrombosis;Pulmonary tumour thrombotic microangiopathy;Pulmonary vasculitis;Pulmonary veno-occlusive disease;Pulmonary venous thrombosis;Pyoderma gangrenosum;Pyostomatitis vegetans;Pyrexia;Quarantine;Radiation leukopenia;Radiculitis 090177e196ea1800\Approved\Approved On: 30-A pr-2021 09:26 (GMT) FDA-CBER-2021-5683-0000089 BNT162b2 5.3.6 Cumulative Analysis of Post-authorization Adverse Event Reports CONFIDENTIAL brachial;Radiologically isolated syndrome;Rash;Rash erythematous;Rash pruritic;Rasmussen encephalitis;Raynaud's phenomenon;Reactive capillary endothelial proliferation;Relapsing multiple sclerosis;Relapsing-remitting multiple sclerosis;Renal amyloidosis;Renal arteritis;Renal artery thrombosis;Renal embolism;Renal failure;Renal vascular thrombosis;Renal vasculitis;Renal vein embolism;Renal vein thrombosis;Respiratory arrest;Respiratory disorder;Respiratory distress;Respiratory failure;Respiratory paralysis;Respiratory syncytial virus bronchiolitis; Respiratory syncytial virus bronchitis;Retinal artery embolism;Retinal artery occlusion; Retinal artery thrombosis;Retinal vascular thrombosis;Retinal vasculitis;Retinal vein occlusion;Retinal vein thrombosis;Retinol binding protein decreased;Retinopathy; Retrograde portal vein flow;Retroperitoneal fibrosis;Reversible airways obstruction; Reynold's syndrome;Rheumatic brain disease;Rheumatic disorder;Rheumatoid arthritis; Rheumatoid factor increased;Rheumatoid factor positive;Rheumatoid factor quantitative increased;Rheumatoid lung;Rheumatoid neutrophilic dermatosis;Rheumatoid nodule;Rheumatoid nodule removal;Rheumatoid scleritis;Rheumatoid vasculitis; Saccadic eye movement;SAPHO syndrome;Sarcoidosis;SARS-CoV-1 test;SARS-CoV-1 test negative;SARS-CoV-1 test positive;SARS-CoV-2 antibody test;SARS-CoV-2 antibody test negative;SARS-CoV-2 antibody test positive;SARS-CoV-2 carrier;SARS-CoV-2 sepsis;SARS-CoV-2 test;SARSCoV-2 test false negative;SARS-CoV-2 test false positive;SARS-CoV-2 test negative;SARSCoV-2 test positive;SARS-CoV-2 viraemia;Satoyoshi syndrome;Schizencephaly;Scleritis;Sclerodactylia;Scleroderma;Sclerode rma associated digital ulcer;Scleroderma renal crisis;Scleroderma-like reaction;Secondary amyloidosis;Secondary cerebellar degeneration;Secondary progressive multiple sclerosis;Segmented hyalinising vasculitis;Seizure;Seizure anoxic;Seizure cluster; Seizure like phenomena;Seizure prophylaxis;Sensation of foreign body;Septic embolus;Septic pulmonary embolism;Severe acute respiratory syndrome;Severe myoclonic epilepsy of infancy;Shock;Shock symptom;Shrinking lung syndrome;Shunt thrombosis;Silent thyroiditis;Simple partial seizures;Sjogren's syndrome;Skin swelling;SLE arthritis;Smooth muscle antibody positive;Sneezing;Spinal artery embolism;Spinal artery thrombosis; Splenic artery thrombosis;Splenic embolism;Splenic thrombosis;Splenic vein thrombosis;Spondylitis;Spondyloarthropathy;Spontaneous heparin-induced thrombocytopenia syndrome;Status epilepticus;Stevens-Johnson syndrome;Stiff leg syndrome;Stiff person syndrome;Stillbirth;Still's disease;Stoma site thrombosis;Stoma site vasculitis;Stress cardiomyopathy;Stridor;Subacute cutaneous lupus erythematosus;Subacute endocarditis;Subacute inflammatory demyelinating polyneuropathy;Subclavian artery embolism;Subclavian artery thrombosis;Subclavian vein thrombosis;Sudden unexplained death in epilepsy;Superior sagittal sinus thrombosis;Susac's syndrome;Suspected COVID19;Swelling;Swelling face;Swelling of eyelid;Swollen tongue;Sympathetic ophthalmia;Systemic lupus erythematosus;Systemic lupus erythematosus disease activity index abnormal;Systemic lupus erythematosus disease activity index decreased;Systemic lupus erythematosus disease activity index increased;Systemic lupus erythematosus rash;Systemic scleroderma;Systemic sclerosis pulmonary;Tachycardia;Tachypnoea;Takayasu's arteritis;Temporal lobe epilepsy;Terminal ileitis;Testicular autoimmunity;Throat tightness;Thromboangiitis obliterans;Thrombocytopenia;Thrombocytopenic purpura;Thrombo phlebitis;Thrombophlebitis migrans;Thrombophlebitis 090177e196ea1800\Approved\ Approved On: 30-A pr-2021 09:26 (GMT) FDA-CBER-2021-5683-0000090 BNT162b2 5.3.6 Cumulative Analysis of Post-authorization Adverse Event Reports CONFIDENTIAL neonatal;Thrombophlebitis septic;Thrombophlebitis superficial;Thromboplastin antibody positive;Thrombosis;Thrombosis corpora cavernosa;Thrombosis in device;Thrombosis mesenteric vessel;Thrombotic cerebral infarction;Thrombotic microangiopathy;Thrombotic stroke;Thrombotic thrombocytopenic purpura;Thyroid disorder;Thyroid stimulating immunoglobulin increased;Thyroiditis;Tongue amyloidosis;Tongue biting;Tongue oedema;Tonic clonic movements;Tonic convulsion;Tonic posturing;Topectomy;Total bile acids increased;Toxic epidermal necrolysis;Toxic leukoencephalopathy;Toxic oil syndrome;Tracheal obstruction;Tracheal oedema;Tracheobronchitis;Tracheobronchitis mycoplasmal;Tracheobronchitis viral;Transaminases abnormal;Transaminases increased;Transfusion-related alloimmune neutropenia;Transient epileptic amnesia;Transverse sinus thrombosis;Trigeminal nerve paresis;Trigeminal neuralgia;Trigeminal palsy;Truncus coeliacus thrombosis;Tuberous sclerosis complex;Tubulointerstitial nephritis and uveitis syndrome;Tumefactive multiple sclerosis;Tumour embolism;Tumour thrombosis; Type 1 diabetes mellitus;Type I hypersensitivity;Type III immune complex mediated reaction;Uhthoff's phenomenon;Ulcerative keratitis;Ultrasound liver abnormal;Umbilical cord thrombosis;Uncinate fits;Undifferentiated connective tissue disease;Upper airway obstruction;Urine bilirubin increased;Urobilinogen urine decreased;Urobilinogen urine increased;Urticaria;Urticaria papular;Urticarial vasculitis;Uterine rupture;Uveitis;Vaccination site thrombosis;Vaccination site vasculitis;Vagus nerve paralysis;Varicella;Varicella keratitis;Varicella post vaccine;Varicella zoster gastritis;Varicella zoster oesophagitis;Varicella zoster pneumonia;Varicella zoster sepsis;Varicella zoster virus infection;Vasa praevia;Vascular graft thrombosis;Vascular pseudoaneurysm thrombosis;Vascular purpura;Vascular stent thrombosis;Vasculitic rash;Vasculitic ulcer;Vasculitis;Vasculitis gastrointestinal;Vasculitis necrotising;Vena cava embolism;Vena cava thrombosis;Venous intravasation;Venous recanalisation;Venous thrombosis;Venous thrombosis in pregnancy;Venous thrombosis limb;Venous thrombosis neonatal;Vertebral artery thrombosis;Vessel puncture site thrombosis;Visceral venous thrombosis;VIth nerve paralysis;VIth nerve paresis;Vitiligo;Vocal cord paralysis;Vocal cord paresis;Vogt-Koyanagi-Harada disease;Warm type haemolytic anaemia;Wheezing;White nipple sign;XIth nerve paralysis;X-ray hepatobiliary abnormal;Young's syndrome;Zika virus associated Guillain Barre syndrome.

APPENDIX IV

Letter to Baroness Hallett, Chair UK Covid-19 Enquiry
Containing Allegations of Mass Murder and Crimes Against Humanity

Dated: May 2023

FREEDOM OF INFORMATION ACT FOIA 2000 REQUEST FOR ALL DEPARTMENTS LISTED TO PROVIDE THEIR REPORTS CONTAINING THEIR RESEARCH DATA THAT REBUTS AND REFUTES ALL ALLEGATIONS PERTAINING IN THIS BOOK AND IN APPENDIX I

Dear Baroness Hallett,

YOU ARE PLACED ON NOTICE
TO SUBMIT THIS BOOK 'COVID COMPENSATION' and APPENDIX I which contains THE LETTER and REPORT THAT ACCOMPANIES THIS BOOK TO YOUR COVID-19 INQUIRY BY July 2023 AND HAVE THE LISTED RECIPIENTS RESPOND TO ITS CONTENTS BY November 2023

THE RECIPIENT LIST IS PLACED ON NOTICE TO RESPOND TO THE BOOK'S CONTENTS and APPENDIX I
(The book may be purchased widely on-line)

Please receive a copy of the book:

<u>COVID COMPENSATION</u>

RECLAIM YOUR
WEALTH & HEALTH
Lost to "Lockdowns" & "VACCINES"
by
Lawrence Wolfe-Xavier

Corona Accountability (Covid19) 2022

A GLOBAL "COVID" MEDICAL & LAW SELF-HELP GUIDE

This book is compiled from research writings and presentations of some of the finest independent minds in the world in: virology, infectious diseases, pulmonary critical care, immunology, epidemiology, microbiology, medicine, virology, law etc including two Nobel Prize winners Luc Montagnier Nobel Prize in Physiology or Medicine for his discovery of the human immunodeficiency virus, Kary Mullis (inventor of PCR TEST in 1987/1988), and one Nobel prize nominee Dr Zelenko Nobel nominee achieved worldwide prominence for treating "COVID-19" patients with hydroxychloroquine and zinc, finding that mortality dropped 8-fold with use of those two substances. He states that treatment with hydroxychloroquine and zinc within the first 5 days reduces death rates by 85%, Robert F Kennedy nephew of President John F Kennedy (deceased), Dr Reiner Fuellmich International Anti-Corporate Corruption Trial Lawyer (Germany/USA) Cofounder 'Corona Investigative Committee' and Founder 'International Crime Investigative Committee' 'ICIC', Professor John P A Ioannidis, the Most Cited Specialist in the World in his fields of evidence-based medicine, epidemiology, and clinical research, Dr Robert Malone USA: Architect of mRNA Technologies et al.

Luc Montagnier:

*'**These "vaccines" are poisons. They are not real vaccines.** The mRNA allows its message to be transcribed throughout the body, uncontrollably. No one can say for each of us where these messages will go. This is therefore a terrible unknown.'*

Kary Mullis:

'Dr Fauci knows nothing..' [Dr Fauci Chief Medical Advisor to President USA, Director of NIAID, USA]

'It* [PCR test] *does not tell you if you are sick' [It is not a diagnostic tool for anything!]

Dr Zelenko:

'the "COVID"/"Vaccination" procedures are 'Crimes against Humanity' and 1st Degree Murder'.

Robert F Kennedy Jr Attorney at Law USA Big Pharma Trial Attorney USA Nephew of John F Kennedy - past President USA:

'This is a designed human tragedy of Biblical proportions.'

Dr Reiner Fuellmich International Anti-Corporate Corruption Trial Lawyer (Germany/USA) Cofounder 'Corona Investigative Committee' and Founder 'International Crime Investigative Committee' 'ICIC':

'New evidence from USA Government "vaccine" Adverse Event Reporting System 'VAERS' data, shows that Big Pharma is coordinating between their companies, on a rationalised premeditated deliberate basis, the distribution of toxic* [Covid19] *"vaccines" that main and kill people.'

'Mass Murder, Crimes Against Humanity' ["Covid19" paradigm]

'there is and was no coronavirus "pandemic", rather only a long-planned, PCR test "casedemic"' ["casedemic" means a "pandemic" of artificially inflated "Covid19" "cases"]

In consideration of the very serious allegations made by these world-wide and world-renowned experts **CORONA ACCOUNTABILITY (Covid19) 2022** formally requests that the entire contents of this book are comprehensively studied by your **Covid-19 Enquiry** and presented to Boris Johnson et al on the distribution list below. Boris Johnson, Matt Hancock, Sajid Javid, Suella Braverman (Attorney General) and Nadhim Zahawi have been sent copies.

Some of the contributors have already agreed to sign sworn oaths as per the UK legal system. We have every confidence that all of them will do so and will be very willing to send their sworn oaths in writing to any UK court that requests them.

We strongly emphasise that these persons are <u>**world leaders**</u> in the most appropriate fields of expertise and that are not mere day-paid journeymen for such organisations as GMC, MHRA, NHS, SAGE, CABINET OFFICE, etc.

Furthermore, if these most eminent persons - mentioned above, peer reviewed study results and data backed allegations, as detailed in this book, are not included in your **Covid-19 Enquiry** report then you, may personally be held to account, for aiding and abetting ***'Mass Murder, Crimes Against Humanity'*** – see above.

THE RECIPIENT LIST IS PLACED ON NOTICE

Letter only to Distribution List:
cc.

<u>**Recipient**</u>	**Office** (at the time – 2019/2020 onwards)
Boris Johnson	**Prime Minister** (copy of book sent)
Matt Hancock	**Health & Social Care** (copy of book sent)
Nadhim Zahawi	**"Covid" "Vaccine" Deployment** (copy of book sent)
Michael Gove	**Cabinet Office**
Sajid Javid	**Health & Social Care** (copy of book sent)
Suella Braverman	**Attorney General** (copy of book sent)
Priti Patel	**Home Office**
Baroness Hallett	**Chair Covid Inquiry 2021-** (principal addressee)
Christopher Whitty	**Chief Medical Officer/Chief Medical Advisor**
Patrick Vallance	**Chief Scientific Advisor**
June Munro Raine	**CEO MHRA** - Medicines and Healthcare Products Regulatory Agency
Charlie Massey	**CEO GMC** – General Medical Council
Amanda Pritchard	**CEO NHS** – National Health Service
Neil Ferguson	**Researcher** - Imperial College, London

Further recipients:

Editors:

John Witherow 'The Times', Chris Evans 'The Telegraph', Ian Hislop 'Private Eye'.

These further recipients may also be personally liable for complicity in ***'Mass Murder, Crimes Against Humanity'*** – as above.

Yours sincerely,

Lawrence Wolfe-Xavier

Editor for:
CORONA ACCOUNTABILITY (Covid19) 2022 27th February 2023
https://covid19compensation2022.com/

Email: corona-accountability-covid19-2022@protonmail.com

LEGAL NOTICE

The contents of the website above, i.e. https://covid19compensation2022.com/, contains material that may be used in **forthcoming criminal prosecutions worldwide**. Any persons or organisations tampering with the website, the website content or its third-party URL links and their content may be liable to prosecution for interfering with criminal case evidence. This Notice is addressed to all persons including Big Tech Companies such as Google, Facebook, Twitter et al.

APPENDIX V

Four pages of Court Documents in Patrick King v Deena Hinshaw, July 2021 Alberta Canada legal case, with particular refence to Schedule A - Request for proof of truly scientific isolation of "SarsCov2" by the isolation of the "virus" from a sample taken from a diseased patient.

COURT FILE NUMBER	2110 00751
COURT	COURT OF QUEEN'S BENCH OF ALBERTA
JUDICIAL CENTRE	RED DEER
APPLICANT	DEENA HINSHAW
RESPONDENT	PATRICK JAMES KING
DOCUMENT	**AFFIDAVIT**
ADDRESS FOR SERVICE AND CONTACT INFORMATION OF PARTY FILING THIS DOCUMENT	ALBERTA JUSTICE CIVIL LITIGATION #1710 639 5th Avenue SW Calgary, Alberta T2P 0M9 TELEPHONE: 403-297-2001 FACSIMILE: 403-662-3824 Cynthia R. Hykaway OUR FILE: LIT- 11840

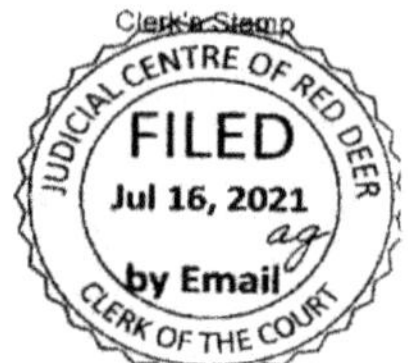

AFFIDAVIT OF KRISZTINA GRECH

Sworn on July 16, 2021

I, Krisztina Grech, of the City of Calgary, in the Province of Alberta, MAKE OATH AND SWEAR THAT:

1. I am employed with the Minister of Justice and Solicitor General for Alberta as a Paralegal in the Legal Services Division. As such, I have personal knowledge of the facts and matters in this Affidavit, except those made on information and belief, in which case I believe them to be true.

2. I am informed by my review of the file, and believe that **Exhibit "A"** to my affidavit is a copy of a Subpoena to a Witness in Provincial Court action number A87988036R that was served on our office on July 15, 2021.

3. I am informed by my review of the file, and believe that **Exhibit "B"** to my affidavit is a copy of the JOIN search of the Respondent, Patrick James King in Provincial Court action number A87988036R.

4. I am informed by my review of the file, and believe that **Exhibit "C"** to my Affidavit a copy of a Violation Ticket issued in in Provincial Court action number A87988036R.

001

5. I am informed by my review of the file, and believe that **Exhibit "D"** to my affidavit a copy of a transcript from May 4, 2021 in Provincial Court action number A87988036R.

SWORN BEFORE ME at the City of Calgary, in the Province of Alberta, this 16th day of July, 2021.

A Commissioner for Oaths in and for the Province of Alberta

CHRISTOPHER GHESQUIERE
BARRISTER AND SOLICITOR

Krisztina Grech

ALBERTA

Subpoena to a Witness
Assignation à un témoin

File/Ticket No. *N° de dossier*: A87988036R

Form 16 — *Formule 16*
Criminal Code Section 699 — *Code criminel Article 699*

Insert full name, residence and occupation of witness. / Insérer le nom complet, le domicile et la profession ou l'occupation du témoin

To / *À* Deena Hinshaw MD
Chief Medical Officer of Health of Alberta
10025 Jasper Ave NW
PO Box 1360 Stn Main
Edmonton, Alberta T5J 2N3

State the offence as in the information. / Indiquer l'infraction comme dans la dénonciation

WHEREAS / *ATTENDU QUE* Patrick James King has been charged that / *a été inculpé d'avoir*
Under Section 73(1) of the Public Health Act – Individual contravening order of medical officer of health

Prosecution or Defence / La poursuite ou la défense

and it has been made to appear that you are likely to give material evidence for the Defence
et qu'on a donné à entendre que vous êtes probablement en état de rendre un témoignage essentiel pour

Set out Court or Justice / Indiquer le tribunal ou le juge de paix

THIS IS THEREFORE TO COMMAND YOU to attend before a Judge
À CES CAUSES, LES PRÉSENTES ONT POUR OBJET DE VOUS ENJOINDRE de comparaître devant
on / *le* 21st day of July 2021 at / *à* 9:30 am
at / *à* Red Deer Provincial Courthouse

to give evidence concerning the said charge, and to bring with you anything in your possession or under your control that relates to the said charge, and more particularly the following:
pour témoigner au sujet de ladite inculpation et d'apporter avec vous toute chose en votre possession ou sous votre contrôle qui se rattachent à ladite inculpation, et en particulier les suivantes:

Specify any documents, objects or other things required / Indiquer les documents, les objets ou autres choses requises

See Attached 'Schedule A'

DATED / *FAIT le* 14 July 2021
at / *à* Red Deer, Alberta
(Seal if required) (*Sceau, s'il est requis*)

KARI CUMMINGS
Justice of the Peace
in and for the Province of Alberta
My Commission Does Not Expire
Juge de paix ou Greffier du tribunal

NOTICE TO WITNESSES: You must report with this Subpoena to the Court Office each day you are required to attend the above hearing and have your attendance recorded thereon. Please arrive a few minutes early to clear Law Courts security.
AVIS AUX TÉMOINS: *Vous devez vous présenter au greffe du tribunal munis de cette assignation chaque jour où vous êtes requis d'être présents à l'audience ci-dessus et y faire consigner votre présence. Veuillez arriver quelques minutes à l'avance pour assurer l'accès sécuritaire au Palais de justice*

CTS0360 (2008/06)

Page 1 of 3

THIS IS EXHIBIT " A "
referred to in the Affidavit of
Krisztina Grech
Sworn before me this 16th
day of July 2021
A Commissioner in and for the Province of Alberta

CHRISTOPHER GHESQUIERE
BARRISTER AND SOLICITOR

To whom it concerns, 'Schedule A'

I request all white papers describing the isolation of the COVID-19 aka SARS-CoV-2 virus in human beings, directly from a sample taken from a diseased patient, where the patient sample was not first combined with any other source of genetic material.

Note: The word "isolate" indicates: a thing is separated from all other material surrounding it.

I am not requesting white papers where "isolation" of SARS-CoV-2 refers to:

- the culturing of something, or

- the performance of an amplification test (PCR), or

- the sequencing of something

To clarify I am requesting via disclosure all white papers showing isolation of the SARS-CoV-2 virus in human beings in your possession or in the possession of Alberta Health ministry, as these white papers would have been integral in the crafting of the statutes made under the "Public Health Act" here in Alberta.

INDEX

D

F

J

O

S

T

Y

Z

M